A History of
Chinese Medicine

A History of Chinese Medicine

DOMINIQUE HOIZEY
and
MARIE-JOSEPH HOIZEY

Translated by
PAUL BAILEY

EDINBURGH UNIVERSITY PRESS

© Editions Payot, 1988

This edition published 1993 by
Edinburgh University Press Ltd
22 George Square, Edinburgh

Typeset in Alphacomp Vladimir
by Pioneer Associates Ltd, Aberfeldy, and
printed in Great Britain by
Hartnoll Ltd, Bodmin

A CIP record for this book is
available from the British Library

ISBN 0 7486 0419 7 (Cased)

ISBN 0 7486 0429 4 (Limp)

Contents

Contents

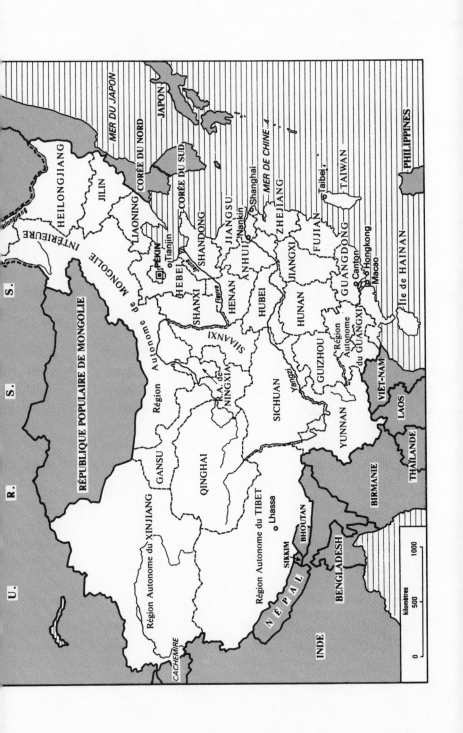

Introduction

Voltaire, who acknowledged the efficacy of Chinese medicine, would, no doubt, have been fascinated by the character of Lady White, half-serpent, half-female, who ran an apothecary known as the Temple of Preserved Harmony. The drugs, ointments and other medicinal wonders scrupulously prepared and generously distributed by the heroine of the legend of the White Serpent vanquished an epidemic as well as the quackery of a malevolent and greedy monk:

Xu, the immortal, and Lady White went to Zhenjiang, where they opened a pharmacy in Number 5 Street called the Temple of Preserved Harmony. At this time, an epidemic was raging in Zhenjiang. Those affected had yellowing complexions, atrophied muscles and extremely low morale. They could be seen everywhere, some laid out on their beds, others stretched out in the streets.

One day, Xu remarked to the White Serpent in a grieved tone: 'Outside an epidemic is raging. Medicine is needed but we no longer have sufficient in the shop. What is to be done?' After reflecting a moment, the White Serpent replied: 'Medicinal plants are the answer, and that's something I know about! Since we will soon run out of medicine, I shall go into the mountains tomorrow and collect plants. As soon as we have such a cure, the people will be saved.' 'There are plenty of savage beasts in the mountains', advised Xu, 'so you need to be careful.' The White Serpent acknowledged Xu's warning, and the next day, at the third hour of the fifth watch and with a basket on her back, she departed on her quest to find medicinal plants. Thirty *li*[1] from the Western Gate, there was a steep mountain known as the Mountain of a Hundred Plants. It was said that in previous times an immense sea had existed there. On an island in this sea were to be found snakes and scorpions

1

everywhere, causing the inhabitants unbearable anxiety throughout the day. The Immortal of the Hundred Plants equipped a boat with medicinal plants and sent it to the island in aid of the unlucky families. He did not anticipate that a fierce wind would blow, which capsized the boat and transformed it into a mountain. Even to this day, the mountain resembles a boat whose hull is pointed towards the sky. All kinds of medicinal plants grew there.

Lady White, perched on a white cloud, flew in the direction of the Mountain of a Hundred Plants. Once there, she hastened to fill her basket to overflowing with medicinal plants such as gentian, honeysuckle and fern, which were then hoarded in the Temple of Preserved Harmony. At the entrance to the pharmacy, Lady White and Xu the immortal displayed on a round table large and small jars into which they poured a medical concoction which was freely offered to everyone. Many lives were thereby saved.

It is commonly said that felicitous events become known 1,000 *li* away. The news spread quickly throughout Zhenjiang that medicine from the Temple of Preserved Harmony performed miracles, and the sick all rushed there. The old monk, Fa Hai, from the Temple of the Gold Mountain, took great offence at this since the sick had previously always come to ask him to devise charms and recite incantations for their illnesses. For the smallest so-called 'miraculous' pill or other cure claimed to be 'supernatural', such people were obliged to offer incense and money. But now they were rushing to the Temple of Preserved Harmony, which meant that the monk would no longer receive incense and money. No wonder he was full of resentment. He enquired further about the situation, and, when he discovered that Lady White was at the centre of it, he felt an even more intense dislike of her. Closing his eyes, he began to think of a plan . . .[2]

The history of Chinese popular religion is replete with monks or Daoist priests who sold written talismans, charms and spells to the ordinary people. According to Father H. Doré, whose *Manuel des Superstitions Chinoises* (1926) noted that 'there were also monks and sorcerers, claiming to be divinely inspired, who recommended preposterous remedies without knowing anything about medicine',[3] these written charms and spells were 'hung outside doors and on household rafters, walls and everyday utensils'. Throughout the history of Chinese medicine, physicians such as Li Shizhen in the sixteenth century railed against medical charlatans and quacks. Even before the shaping of the principles on which Chinese medicine was based more than 2,000 years ago, the Chinese often appealed to faith-healing sorcerers. It is thus no coincidence that the written character for 'sorcerer' (*wu*) forms part of the character *yi*, which refers to the skill of curing as well as to the person who exercises such a skill.

During the Spring and Autumn period (770–476 BC), the Chinese world underwent fundamental change. Theories of the *yin* and the *yang* and of the five elements made their appearance, providing the basis for a newly-developing medicine and an answer to the question posed by the Yellow Emperor: 'Why do people nowadays not live to 100 years?'

This history of Chinese medicine from prehistoric times to the present begins with myth, legend and belief. This is not solely because they impart fascinating yarns but also, as Claude Lévi-Strauss has noted, because

> the principal value of myths and rites is to preserve until the present time the remains of methods of observation and reflection which were (and no doubt still are) precisely adapted to discoveries of a certain type: those which nature sanctioned from the starting point of a speculative organization and exploitation of the perceptible world in terms of perception. This science of the concrete was necessarily restricted by its essence to results other than those destined to be achieved by the exact natural sciences, but it was no less scientific and its results no less genuine. Those results, having been affirmed ten thousand years before others, still underpin our own civilization.[4]

To control illness is a long-standing desire of humankind, and it was probably with some trepidation that during the Shang dynasty (1766–1122 BC) shamans were often asked to consult the ancestors on an imminent birth, what course a headache might take, or even (3,000 years before Freud) the significance of a dream. The earliest origins of medicine in China can be dated from this period. I shall examine the evolution of Chinese medicine as it developed during the course of dynastic history, without overlooking the principal aims and concrete results of the politics of health pursued after 1949 by the People's Republic, the inheritor of a long tradition of health care.

I have principally used Chinese sources, in particular Yu Shenchu, *Zhongguo Yixue Jianshi* (*A Concise History of Chinese Medicine*,

Fuzhou: Fujian Kexue Jishu Chubanshe, 1983); Zhen Zhiya, *Zhongguo Yixueshi* (*A History of Chinese Medicine*, Shanghai: Shanghai Kexue Jishu Chubanshe, 1984, 1985); Fan Xingzhun, *Zhongguo Yixue Shilue* (*A Brief History of Chinese Medicine*, Beijing: Zhongyi Guji Chubanshe, 1986); Jia Weicheng, *Sanbai Zhong Yiji Lu* (*Catalogue of 300 Books on Chinese Medicine*, Harbin: Heilongjiang Kexue Jishu Chubanshe, 1982); Li Xiangzhong, *Zhongguo Yixue Jichu* (*The Essential Book of Chinese Medicine*, Beijing: Renmin Weisheng Chubanshe, 1978, 1984); *Quanguo Zhongcaoyao Huibian* (*National Catalogue of Chinese Medicinal Herbs*, Beijing: Renmin Weisheng Chubanshe, 1975, 1983); *Zhongyaozhi* (*Monograph on Chinese Medicine*, Beijing: Renmin Weisheng Chubanshe, 1959, 1982); *Chinese-English Glossary of Common Terms in Traditional Chinese Medicine* (Guangzhou: Guangdong Keji Chubanshe, 1982); and *Zhonghua Yishi Zazhi* (*Chinese Journal of Medical History*). I have not thought it necessary to give a more extensive bibliography; the books and articles directly related to this study are, of course, referred to in the footnotes. On the other hand, I have added a number of appendices, notably a chronological table outlining the history of Chinese medicine, as well as indexes of persons and plants cited in the text.

Notes

1. One *li* is equivalent to half a kilometre.
2. Author's translation of the version given in *Zhenjiang Minjian Gushi* (Beijing: Zhongguo Minjian Wenyi Chubanshe, 1982).
3. H. Doré, *Manuel des Superstitions Chinoises* (Paris: Centre de publication de l'UER Extrême-Orient-Asie du Sud-Est, 1970), pp 35–45.
4. Claude Lévi-Strauss, *The Savage Mind* (London: Weidenfeld and Nicholson, 1966), p 16.

— 1 —

From Mythology to History

In the Beginning was the Myth

The history of Chinese medicine begins with a myth. Legend recounts that the Yellow Emperor (*Huangdi*) asserted himself as the supreme ruler of the universe. He occupied the centre, leaving the south to the Fire Emperor (*Yandi*), sometimes known as the Red Emperor, who was said to have the body of a man but the head of a bull. The Fire Emperor's sense of benevolence prompted him to teach men how to cultivate the five grains (i.e. millet, rye, sesame and two kinds of wheat), which has earned him the title of the Divine Farmer (*Shen'nong*). He possessed a magic whisk which was used to discover whether a plant was poisonous or not and to determine the nature of such a plant. If the case arose, therefore, the Fire Emperor could offer a prescription to treat various illnesses. He would even taste a plant himself to examine its effects, since his transparent body allowed him to neutralise any poisonous matter inadvertently taken by rubbing the appropriate herb on the affected part of his body. The day finally came, however, when the poison got the better of his skill.

The Fire Emperor's rival, the Yellow Emperor, was also attributed with therapeutic skills. In fact, most things were attributed to the Yellow Emperor and his ministers, ranging from the pestle and mortar to the bow, chariot, boat, mirror, drum and even the musical and mathematical scales. It was one of these ministers, Wu Peng, who pioneered the art of medicine. Chinese tradition also mentions the names of three physicians who lived during this mythical age: Yu Fu, who distinguished himself as a surgeon, Lei Gong, and Qi Bo.[1] Whatever the historical validity of the Yellow Emperor and the Fire Emperor and of their scientific skills, both have given their names to two medical works, the *Huangdi Neijing* (Yellow Emperor's *Classic of Internal Medicine*) and the *Shen'nong*

5

Bencaojing (*Classic of Herbal Medicine*), which will be analysed later.

The *Huangdi Neijing* begins with a question put by the Yellow Emperor to his physician, Qi Bo: 'I have heard that in ancient times people lived 100 years, yet today they only live fifty years. Why is the present situation so different?' Qi Bo replied that men in ancient times took as their models the *yin* and the *yang*, ensuring that the spirit (*yang*) and the body (*yin*) were in perfect harmony. Man could not escape, he continued, the universal law of the *yin* and the *yang*, and his health depended on the equilibrium of these two opposing forces. An excess of one or a diminution of the other could engender sickness. On the other hand, as the author of the Daoist classic, *Lie zi*, was to point out, when the *yin* and the *yang* are in perfect harmony, 'care and sustenance will surely come in their time, the annual harvest will always be plentiful, people will never experience illness and die prematurely, and demons shall never appear'.[2]

Humankind did not have to wait for Schopenhauer before discovering that suffering is omnipresent. Since the very beginning, humans have persistently sought to divest themselves of this undesirable companion that has haunted their lives. Myths, legends and folklore all attest to man's anguish and sense of impotence in the face of disease, which, despite everything, he has always tried to prevent. Man has also been content to tell of the assistance provided by benevolent gods in this quest, as the following Manchu tale from the north-east shows.

The god Abukasiduli sent Sidulizengtu to earth as the protector of humanity, thus arousing the jealousy of Yeluli, who resolved to bring harm to humankind. Abukasiduli thereupon ordered Duolong-beizi to kill Yeluli. Yeluli's soul, with nowhere to go, finally created a hell in which to reside. Vowing to destroy humanity, Yeluli brought pestilence to the land. On hearing the people's cry for help, Abukasiduli sent the god Nandanweihuli, whose stomach, in appearance like that of humans, was quite transparent so that all its internal organs were visible. In order to rescue suffering humanity, Nandanweihuli collected and tasted various medicinal plants, soon discovering ways of treating smallpox, fevers and chills. He prepared a number of effective remedies and gathered disciples around him. The epidemic was soon eliminated. Yeluli, however, planted seven poisonous plants in secret, one of which Nandanweihuli tasted inadvertently one day. Before long, he felt pain in his stomach, and, looking down, noticed that the poison was already attacking the liver. Enduring the agony, and knowing he did not have long to live, Nandanweihuli searched for the poisonous plants. He discovered six of them, which he consumed himself. The poison gradually spread throughout his entire body but, on the point of death, he was able to warn his disciples of the potential harm that the seventh plant could bring.[3]

Chinese folklore, particularly that of ethnic minorities, is rich with legends that testify to man's concern with illness. Thus the Elunchun, who live in the northern province of Heilongjiang, have preserved the memory of three deities who guard humankind against smallpox ('heavenly flowers' in Chinese), measles and fever.[4] In southern China, the Dai people of Yunnan province tell the story of a physician's granddaughter who set out to discover a miraculous lotus flower that would combat a local epidemic. On returning from her journey, the young girl was transformed into a lotus whose blossom was red with her blood. It was believed that after this the Dai people 'once again led happy lives'.[5] More often, legends might refer to various medicinal plants without going into details on their therapeutic value. The Dai legend of the 'dragon's tongue' (*Agave americana*), for example, simply mentions at the end of the tale that it was used to cure sickness, but the story itself is not directly concerned with the plant's properties.[6]

By way of contrast, the Bai, another minority living in the south, recount the extraordinary origins of the Chinese angelica (*Angelica sinensis*), called *dang'gui* in Chinese, and detail the benefits of this 'invigorating' plant:

> There were once two brothers from a poor family. The idleness of the elder was matched only by the diligence of the younger. After the death of their parents, the elder brother expelled his younger brother from the home and took sole possession of the family property. The younger brother was left with only a bow and some arrows their father had used for hunting.

> From that time on, the younger brother, his bow slung across his back, spent his days hunting. One day, he noticed a falcon resting on a huge chestnut tree. As he took aim at the bird, it spoke to him in human language, appealing to his good nature and begging him not to fire the arrow. 'My mother', the falcon explained, 'is blind and has need of me to provide food. If you let me go, I shall give you some seeds of medicinal herbs.' The younger brother put away his bow and replied: 'Poor falcon, I will not kill you but I do not need your gift. Go quickly and find food for your mother.' The falcon thereupon spat a drop of blood containing the seeds of medicinal herbs, and flew away. The brother picked up a few of the seeds and returned to his

hut. He planted them in a plot of ground facing the sun in front of his hut. Three days later, young shoots appeared, and three days after that they had become sturdy stems. Small flowers as red as blood blossomed. He broke off a root and ate it, whereupon his appearance became robust and his whole being invigorated. He gave roots to the villagers to eat, and those who had been ill were immediately cured while those who had not been ill gained renewed strength. On that day, small birds with red plumage and golden beaks flew around the roof of the brother's hut screeching ceaselessly 'dang'gui, dang'gui'. Thus the medicinal plant was called *dang'gui*.[7]

The Chinese angelica grows principally in the provinces of Gansu, Ningxia, Yunnan and Sichuan. The most celebrated is the one that grows in the district of Min in Gansu. It is often said that 'the Chinese angelica is the best in the world, but that of Min is the best in China'. It has been used for gynaecological purposes for a long time, since the *Classic of Herbal Medicine*, a work dating from the first years of the Christian era, recommends this plant to cure period pains.

The Chinese angelica is not the only medicinal plant to have inspired the imagination of storytellers. Ginseng, as well as gingko, have their own mythology, but less prestigious plants also have their folklore. Such plants include the 'heavenly hemp' (*Gastrodia elata*), whose rootstock is used in traditional Chinese medicine to lower blood pressure and to cure dizzy spells and headaches, the multiflowered polygonum (*Polygonum multiflorum*), valued for its treatment of anaemia, insomnia and neurasthenia, and the artemisia, celebrated in a Bai folktale as an anodyne to soothe painful nettle-stings.

This Bai folktale tells the story of two abandoned sisters who fell into the clutches of an ogress. One sister was eaten, but the other escaped and hid in a tree. Although she succeeded in killing the ogress, the latter was transformed into nettles on the point of death, thus preventing the young girl from climbing down the tree. A cowherd refused to help her and she had to appeal to some shepherds, who threw a woollen quilt over the nettles. The unfortunate girl fell awkwardly in the midst of the nettles and was transformed into a beautiful artemisia. The story concludes that 'since then, whenever one is stung by a nettle, all one needs to do is to rub oneself with an artemisia to soothe the pain'.[8]

In China, the artemisia has a long medical tradition, and it is virtually synonymous with moxibustion. This therapeutic process consists of cauterising certain chosen parts of the body with powder and burning artemisia leaves (*Artemisia vulgaris*). The plant has been highly valued not only by therapists and patients but also by poets, since one can find in the Classic of Odes (*Shijing*), the earliest anthology of Chinese poems, the following lines:

> How majestic the artemisia
> Enveloped by dewdrops.

A Perusal of the *Classic of Mountains and Seas*

In his study of the *Classic of Mountains and Seas* (*Shanhaijing*), Rémi Mathieu writes: 'At the dawn of a people's history there often occurs an understanding of the things of nature which seems to compensate for an ignorance of the nature of things'.[9] The *Classic of Mountains and Seas*, famous for the myths it records, is an extraordinary work of ancient China. It distils the knowledge of an entire era, that of the Han (206 BC – 220 AD), and is a kind of proto-encyclopaedia in the fields of botany, zoology, geology and medicine. Concerning the latter, a few extracts from Mathieu's translation can be cited:

> Eighty *li* further west is Mount Fuyu. On its southern slope there is an abundance of copper, on its northern slope there is an abundance of iron; on the peak there grows a tree called *wenheng*. Its fruit resembles the jujube and is eaten to alleviate deafness. As for plants there are many shaddocks. They resemble the wild mallow but have red blossoms and yellow fruit. Their leaves look like a child's tongue. Whoever eats the fruit can avoid mental disorder.

> Dwarf fig-trees can be seen . . . whoever eats the figs can cure his heart problems.

> 360 *li* to the south-west is Mount Yanzi. On its summit there are many cinnabar-red trees. Their leaves resemble those of the Chinese mulberry and their fruit are as large as gourds. They have red stalks and black veins, and whoever eats such fruit can be cured of jaundice.

From a reading of the *Classic of Mountains and Seas*, one could almost devise a prescription handbook for medical emergencies. Thus for stomach-ache it is recommended to eat the petaurist. The flesh of this 'flying squirrel' will soothe the pain, but if it is a question of indigestion then it is better to eat a strange bird which has 'four wings, one eye and the tail of a dog' and whose cry 'resembles that of a magpie'. To combat flatulence, one could eat a fish 'whose odour is similar to the scent of a lovage', while haemorrhoids could be dealt with by eating the flesh of the 'crocodile-tiger'. The fruit of the 'thistle-cypress' helps resistance against the cold, and the meat of the small horned owl cures sunstroke. For headache, one could always eat heron. If one is tired, there are plenty of options, but what is recommended is the tree whose fruit 'resembles peaches' and whose leaves 'resemble those of the jujube'. If you have to scratch yourself, bathing with the 'white blossom' of the asclepias (milkweed) will get rid of the itching and boils.

One could cite further examples and thus learn that on Mount Beihao there are trees whose fruit 'prevents malaria', or that on Mount Tuohu there is a plant whose fruit 'cures ophthalmia'. It is well known that China is particularly well endowed with edible fruits. Ming Wong notes that 'botanists have singled out more than 300 kinds, divided principally into two categories: dry fruit (pods, capsules, achenes) and fleshy fruit (stone-fruit, berries), sought after by both gastronomes and pharmacists'.[10] One also learns from the *Classic of Mountains and Seas* of the tree 'whose fruit resembles that of the eupatorium (hemp agrimony); when a woman eats it, she will not become pregnant'. One might ask, with Rémi Mathieu, whether this is describing a contraceptive method or is simply an aetiological explanation of sterility. It is not the only plant mentioned in the *Classic of Mountains and Seas* that is said to cause sterility. Thus mention is also made of the plant 'whose leaves resemble those of the basil' and whose root 'is similar to that of the platycodon (balloon-flower)'.

Whatever the case, the *Classic of Mountains and Seas*, the first chapters of which probably antedate the Qin unification of 221 BC, astounds the contemporary reader with its knowledge of plants known to have therapeutic value. The description of the scopolia (*solanacaea*) is particularly noteworthy: 'A plant is to be found there which resembles the achillea but which has green downy leaves and white fruit, and is called the scopolia. When taken, it can prevent premature death and help to cure stomach ailments.' Today, in traditional Chinese medicine, *scopolia tangutica* is recommended for the treatment of chronic or acute gastritis and enteritis. The asclepias (milkweed), which, according to the *Classic of Mountains and Seas*, is well-known for its healing of itches and boils, is recognised in China by the name of *luomo* (*Metaplexis japonica*). It has a white blossom, and its root is used in the treatment of asthenia and sexual impotence; and, indeed, it is also externally used in the healing of boils.

Louis Lewin, to whom we owe the first clinical classification of drugs, writes:

> From the moment man first appeared in the mists of history, he became addicted to certain substances, not because of the need for nourishment but in order to achieve, whenever he felt the urge, a momentary state of euphoria and ease which would give him the feeling of subjective well-being.[11]

It is therefore not surprising to find in the *Classic of Mountains and Seas* references to several mind-affecting drugs, 'the supply of which', as Claude Meyers reminds us in his *Histoire des drogues et médicaments de l'esprit*, 'was already available in antiquity and which greatly expanded shortly thereafter with the appearance of synthetic products'.[12] Rather than drugs per se, the *Classic of Mountains and Seas* refers more to remedies that have narcotic effects, such as a wild cat which, 'if reared ... can help cure melancholy'. The question is whether it is the cat's company or its meat that is the antidepressant. There is also a reference to small sturgeons with the 'head of a dog' whose meat cures insanity. One can avert anger by adorning oneself with the flowers or fruit of a tree called 'emperor's rest'; one can avoid muddle-headedness by wearing on one's belt the blossom of a tree akin to the Chinese mulberry. The most bizarre of these remedies is no doubt the flesh of the oriole, which 'cures jealousy'.

The Long Birthpangs of Chinese Medicine: From Early Man in China to the 'Cultural Revolution' of the New Stone Age

From Yuanmou man,[13] who appeared 1,700,000 years ago, to the neolithic era (via the celebrated Beijing man, who Pierre Teilhard de Chardin in 1937 argued should be regarded 'as a being in whom the flame of reflective thought had already, and doubtless for a long time before, been lit'[14]) stretched an 'immense time-span characterised by a gradual process of pathbreaking experiment and change'.[15] Included in this process were the first stumblings of an empirical medicine that first developed out of contact with the animal, vegetable and mineral worlds. As we have seen, the *Classic of Mountains and Seas* provides numerous examples: the flesh of a certain animal 'prevents furunculosis'; the fruit of a certain tree 'prevents malaria'. Prehistoric man, living off wild fruit, seeds and roots, discovered that what he ingested could provoke vomiting, diarrhoea, fainting and even death. More than this, writes Yu Shenchu, a historian of Chinese medicine, 'after innumerable and repeated experiments, man gradually learnt to recognise the properties of plants and began to use them specifically to deal with certain illnesses'.[16]

What evidence remains of this period of experiment? The long and gradual progress of the first man in China, from early to later palaeolithic times, has left little trace of any medical practice. Beijing man, who lived 200,000–500,000 years ago, fed on small animals such as rats and frogs, numerous fossils of which can be found in ash deposits. No doubt he also gathered wild fruit. Nettle seeds (*Celtis bungeana*) have been recovered, but 'this is all that remains', writes Jia Lanpo, 'as proof of a partially vegetarian diet'.[17] Although Beijing man, as Pierre Teilhard de Chardin succinctly remarked, had crossed over 'the mysterious threshold separating instinct from reflection'[18] (he was able to work skilfully with flint, sandstone and quartz), did he know how to treat a wound? How did Dali man,[19] who lived 100,000–200,000 years ago, react in the face of illness? How did people of Dingcun, Changyang, Maba or Xujiayao,[20] who belong to the middle palaeolithic era, behave in the wake of an epidemic? The sole objects left by these people are their stone tools. What Denise de Donneville-Bordes has observed of man during the middle palaeolithic era in Europe is equally valid for his Chinese contemporary, that is he had at his active disposal 'a significant body of attainment which revealed an advance towards the mental and cultural outlook by means of which his successor would accomplish a giant stride forward in kind'.[21] Xujiayao man, for example, who lived 30,000–60,000 years ago, represents morphologically a distinct stage of evolution in comparison with Beijing man from whom he descended. His tools included carefully-wrought stone chips, blocks, tips and chisels, with their diminutive size being particularly striking. One can in fact detect here the earliest microlithic activity in China, although there is no concrete evidence to show whether Xujiayao man had the means to mitigate pain or cure an illness.

Homo sapiens finally arrived, but again there is the problem of evidence: the culture of the higher palaeolithic era, including that of man of the Zhoukoudian cave (one of the most well-known representative sites in north China at the end of the palaeolithic age), gives no clue as to the origins of Chinese medicine. Exhumed human remains at Zhoukoudian have been closely examined because they reveal various skull wounds. Weidenreich considers the remains as those of a family who were victims of a sudden attack.[22] Other hypotheses have been suggested. It might be that the family was simply interred there following an epidemic. It is equally valid to suppose that the skull wounds were due to a rock-fall after burial.

Whatever the tragic fate of this family (if indeed it was a family), Yu Shenchu refers to one of its members as the victim of a skull wound that might have been caused by some kind of tool.[23] Is this a case of trepanation (perforation of the skull) that prehistorians have suggested occurred at this time? The purpose was perhaps to deliver a patient from a mysterious illness (one could imagine a tumour, for example), but a ritual explanation cannot be excluded.

All evidence shows that, from time immemorial, man has sought to liberate himself from pain. At the beginning, no doubt, he was happy to use saliva, peat, plant-stalks, tree-bark, leaves and moss to dress a wound. Arrow wounds necessitated the use of flint knives, and one can imagine that such knives were at first used to lance abscesses and then gradually utilised for amputation, hysterotomy, castration and even trepanation, which was common in neolithic times. Jean Zammit writes:

> it is very likely that the person performing the trepanation had to use a flint knife, which allowed him to section the scalp and make an incision, all the while moving the skull sideways so as to avoid damaging the membranes and other brain tissue. As this delicate operation required the patient to be absolutely immobile so as to avoid any mortal cut, one might wonder whether plant-derived drugs were not available to ease the pain and keep the patient in a semi-conscious state.[24]

The neolithic or New Stone Age era was characterised not only by the polishing of stone to be used as tools, but also by the practice of agriculture and animal husbandry. A tribal subsistence economy based on gathering and hunting was replaced by a village economy in which man was transformed from a predator to a producer. The scope of this 'cultural revolution' can especially be discerned in the development of ceramics, an activity in which neolithic man demonstrated all his ingenuity and art. This varied development began with the rough pottery of Lijiacun, Laoguantai and Beiligang, communities that existed as long as 7,000–8,000 years ago,[25] and proceeded to the elegant black pottery of Longshan culture (2900–2200 BC). In between came the painted pottery of Yangshao culture (5000–3000 BC), as well as the unique pottery of Dawenkou (4500–2300 BC), notable for the triangular and circular shapes pierced at the base, and the pottery of Majiayao culture (3000–2000 BC), located in Gansu and whose geometrical and spiral designs are particularly noticeable.

The earliest neolithic cultures discovered in China suggest only a slightly developed society, composed of primitive communities and in which agriculture played a modest role. Yangshao culture, on the

other hand, witnessed the cultivation of millet, and it is also quite
likely that the growing of hemp took place. The raising of silkworms
was probably not unknown either, since Yangshao people spun and
wove. The succeeding Longshan culture (it is thought that it replaced
Yangshao culture throughout north China) developed agriculture to
the point that it superseded hunting and fishing in importance. Out
of forty or so tools discovered at twenty-five sites belonging to
Longshan culture, the majority comprises agricultural implements.[26]
At Hemedu, a neolithic site in the province of Zhejiang, rice was
being cultivated as early as 5000 BC.

The evolution of society is clearly shown by Dawenkou culture
during its final phase around 2800–2300 BC. The wealth of funeral
property discovered in certain tombs has prompted Gao Guangren
to comment:

> The question arises whether these craft objects of such variety
> and good quality were specifically made for clan use as a
> whole, or whether they were simply the result of a sideline
> activity amongst an essentially agricultural people. In fact, it
> seems likely that during the last period of the neolithic era a
> stage had been reached whereby certain people detached
> themselves from agricultural work and devoted all their time to
> handicraft production; a handful of noble families, taking
> advantage of their power and prestige within the clan, insisted
> on being the sole recipients of such handicrafts. In this way
> there emerged within the clan itself social inequalities that
> anticipated the system of private property . . .[27]

The neolithic period also witnessed the beginnings of a writing
system, or at least the appearance of what some have confirmed are
definite pictograms, such as those depicting a sun above the clouds
and a sun setting below a mountain which have been engraved on
pottery excavated at two sites belonging to Dawenkou culture.
Earlier pictograms have been discovered on Yangshao pottery,
notably at Jiangzhai.[28]

It was during this period of several millennia that an emerging
Chinese medicine was able to endow itself with certain implements,
such as the 'stones used as needles', referred to in the *Classic of
Mountains and Seas*. Archaeological activity has brought to light a
number of strangely-pointed stones (called *bian* in Chinese), which
the *Shouwen Jiezi*, a dictionary compiled in the Han dynasty,
describes as stone slivers for medical usage; they were used to make
skin incisions. It is virtually certain that acupuncture originated
with the use of these stone, and then bone and bamboo, needles,
which people later learnt to employ for therapeutic purposes.

The Shang Period

The mythical emperors Yao and Shun were succeeded by Yu, the founder of the semi-mythical dynasty of Xia (2205?–1766? BC), which preceded that of the Shang (1766–1122 BC). According to tradition, the last ruler of Xia, the tyrant Jie, was defeated and then exiled by one of his vassals, Cheng Tang. It was Cheng Tang who founded the Shang (or Yin) dynasty, the first of the Bronze Age, and which lasted until the advent of the western Zhou in the eleventh millennium BC. 'On the whole,' observes Jacques Gernet, 'writing, the chariot, architectural techniques, the practice of divination, and the art of working in bronze . . . all appear in the lower basin of the Yellow River in forms that are already very elaborate.' However, he adds, 'it is by its religious practices and their predominant role that the Shang civilization is most clearly distinguished from that of the following age'.[29] Divination by fire, human sacrifice and the ritual worship of deceased kings were the most striking manifestations of these religious practices. The celebrated 'oracle-bone inscriptions' (written on turtle-shells and shoulder-blades of cattle and other animals) have revealed numerous aspects of this ancient monarchy. They refer to a number of activities, from the prospects of a military campaign ('Should the king undertake a military campaign against the barbarians this spring?') to the birth of a child ('Will Lady Hao be in good health after the birth of her baby?'), as well as discussing the construction of a city, hunting and illness ('Will the king suffer from a toothache?').

Archaeology shows that the people of Shang took care of their health. In 1973, at a Shang site in Taixi near the town of Gaocheng (Hubei province), over thirty particles of stone-fruit were discovered, among which were peach and Japanese plum (*Prunus japonica*) stones. It is precisely such fruit stones that have for a long time been appreciated for their therapeutic qualities. The peach-stone is mentioned in *Shen'nong Bencaojing* (*Classic of Herbal Medicine*), where it is especially recommended for 'eliminating tapeworm'. Today, Chinese traditional medicine uses it in gynaecology. The curative efficacy of the Japanese plum-stone was likewise recognised by the authors of *Shen'nong Bencaojing*. The authors of an article published in a Chinese archaeological journal write that 'the discovery of peach and plum-stones originating from the Shang era demonstrates a development of Chinese phytotherapy (treatment with plants or plant extracts) more than 3,000 years ago'.[30]

The Shang site at Taixi offered another surprise for historians of Chinese medicine. A stone 'hook' measuring 20 cm in length and

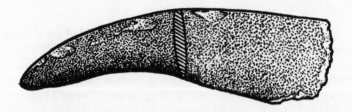

FIGURE 1.1   A stone hook (*bian*) excavated from the Shang site at
Taixi. From *Gaocheng Taixi Shangdai Yizhi* (Beijing: Wenwu
Chubanshe, 1977).

5.4 cm by maximum width was retrieved from one of the excavated
tombs. It was originally contained in a lacquer casket, indicating
that it was not an ordinary tool but rather an object of value. Ma
Jixing observes that 'it was a medical instrument of the time, a kind
of *bian* . . .', the pointed stone that was described earlier. Moreover,
Chinese surgeons have for a long time made use of hook-shaped
instruments. One work dating from 1736 refers to 'large and small
curved knives', while another, in 1907, mentions a 'bent knife'. In
1856, the *Waike Tushuo* (*Illustrated Manual of Surgery*) showed
'curved' knives in 'willow-like' or 'hook-shaped' form. According to
Ma Jixing, all these instruments were derived from the *bian* of
antiquity.[31]

The making of fermented wine, which took place during the
Shang and which has bequeathed magnificent bronzes such as
vases to store the wine and drinking-cups, was not unconnected
with the development of medicine. 'Medicinal wines' soon made an
appearance. The Chinese character *yi*, meaning to 'treat an illness'
(and hence 'medicine'), contains the radical *jiu* which, on its own,
refers to all kinds of alcoholic drink. Thus the oldest Chinese
dictionary, *Shuowen Jiezi*, defines the character *yi* as 'to discharge
arrows' against malevolent influences causing illness by giving the
patient reinvigorating elixirs (*jiu*). The practice of decoction likewise
contributed to the growth of a burgeoning medicine. Finally, it
seems that hygiene was one of the preoccupations of the time, since
some of the oracle-bone inscriptions refer to washing the face,
hands and feet and even to taking a bath. Excavation at Shang sites
has produced various items of personal hygiene such as jade combs
and bronze mirrors, as well as jugs and basins that may have been
used for washing.

Medicine was practised by shaman-healers, indicated by the fact
that one of the pictograms for *yi* (medicine) contains the character

wu (shaman). They combined drugs and incantations to cure scabies and malaria, two afflictions that were current at the time. The *Classic of Mountains and Seas* recounts that ten shamans followed one another in climbing Mount Ling and thereupon 'the hundred kinds of drug were found there'. Another passage refers to the existence of shamans who 'had at hand the plant of immortality'. What Jean-Marie Pelt has written of black African tradition is equally valid for the shaman-healers of the Shang era:

> It was incumbent upon the faith-healer to forge the link between man and powerful occult forces, those 'spirits' that peopled the rich pantheon of animism. It thus fell upon him to undertake the cause of healing sickness, in the process demonstrating the power of his word and hence gaining the appropriate virtue.[32]

Notes

1. See Jan and Yvonne Walls, *Classical Chinese Myths* (Hong Kong: Joint Publishing Co., 1984). For readers of Chinese, a useful reference is Yuan Ke, *Zhongguo Shenhua Chuanshuo* (Beijing: Zhongguo Minjian Wenyi Chubanshe, 1984).
2. See Benedykt Grynpas's translation of the *Liezi* in *Philosophes Taoistes* (Paris: Bibliothèque Pléiade, 1980), p 387.
3. From *Manzu Minjian Gushixuan* (Shanghai: Shanghai Wenyi Chubanshe, 1983).
4. *Elunchunzu Minjian Gushiji* (Beijing: Zhongguo Minjian Wenyi Chubanshe, 1984).
5. See the folklore journal *Shancha*, no 1 (1984).
6. *Daizu Minjian Gushixuan* (Shanghai: Shanghai Wenyi Chubanshe, 1985).
7. *Baizu Minjian Gushixuan* (Shanghai: Shanghai Wenyi Chubanshe, 1984).
8. Ibid.
9. Rémi Mathieu, *Etude sur la Mythologie et l'Ethnologie de la Chine Ancienne* (Paris: Institut des Hautes Etudes Chinoises, 1983). All citations from the *Shanhaijing* are taken from Mathieu's excellent translation.
10. Ming Wong, *La Médecine Chinoise par les Plantes* (Paris, 1976), p 109.
11. Louis Lewin, *Phantastica: Drogue Psychédélique* (Paris: Petite Bibliothèque Payot, 1970).
12. Claude Meyers, *Brève Histoire des Drogues et Médicaments de l'Esprit* (Paris: Editions Erès, 1985).
13. In 1965, two fossilised teeth which are thought to belong to a *Homo erectus* of the Lower Pleistocene period were discovered near Yuanmou, in Yunnan province. On this, see 'Preliminary Study on the Age of Yuanmou Man by Palaeomagnetic Technique', *Scientia Sinica*, 20:5 (September–October 1977).
14. Pierre Teilhard de Chardin, *L'Apparition de l'Homme* (Paris: Editions de Seuil, 1956).
15. Louis-René Nougier, *L'Economie Préhistorique* (Paris: PUF, 1970).

16. Yu Shenchu, *Zhongguo Yixue Jianshi* (Fuzhou: Fujian Kexue Jishu Chubanshe, 1983).
17. Jia Lanpo, *Beijing Caveman* (Beijing: Foreign Language Press, 1978).
18. Pierre Teilhard de Chardin, op. cit.
19. Dominique Hoizey, 'L'Homme de Dali', *Initiation à l'Archéologie et à la Préhistoire* (August 1980).
20. Jia Lanpo, op. cit., notes in connection with the discoveries at Dingcun, in Shanxi province: 'They represent a significant link in the reconstruction of prehistoric culture. Further excavation and analysis have proved that the influence of Dingcun extended throughout the Fen River valley, giving rise to an evolving community more than 100,000 years ago.' See also Michèle Pirazzoli-t' Serstevens, 'Extrême-Orient, Chine: Paléolithique, Néolithique et âge du bronze', in *Encyclopaedia Universalis*, and Kwang-chih Chang, *The Archeology of Ancient China* (New Haven: Yale University Press, 1977).
21. Denise de Sonneville-Bordes, *La Préhistoire Moderne* (Périgueux: Pierre Fanlac, 1972).
22. Kwang-chih Chang, op. cit.
23. Yu Shenchu, op. cit.
24. Jean Zammit, 'L'Homme néolithique et la maladie', *Dossiers de l'Archéologie*, no 44 (June 1980).
25. These cultures were situated in the middle reaches of the Yellow River basin and along the upper reaches of the Han River.
26. Tong Zhuchen, *Longshan Wenhua* (Beijing, 1978).
27. Gao Guangren, 'Prehistoric civilization of Dawenkou', *China Reconstructs* (August 1978). See also an article by the same author in *Kaogu Xuebao*, no 4 (1978).
28. Dominique Hoizey, 'D'où vient l'Ecriture chinoise?', *L'Histoire* (September 1981).
29. Jacques Gernet, *A History of Chinese Civilization* (Cambridge: Cambridge University Press, 1982), pp 41, 45.
30. 'Gaocheng Shangdai yizhizhong chutude taoren he yuliren', *Wenwu*, no 8 (1978).
31. Ma Jixing, 'Taixicun Shangmuzhong chutude yiliao qiju bianlian', *Wenwu*, no 6 (1979).
32. Jean-Marie Pelt, *La Médecine par les Plantes* (Paris: Fayard, 1981).

2

From the Western Zhou to the End of the Warring States Period, 1100–221 BC

Specialists at the Zhou Court

His overriding concern was that the people had sufficient to eat and that the funeral and sacrificial rites were appropriately performed. Through his generosity of spirit and his sincerity he gained the people's support and confidence, while his diligence and justice brought them success and happiness.[1]

With these words, Confucius rendered homage to King Wu, the founder of the Zhou dynasty, usually divided into the Western Zhou (eleventh century to 771 BC) and Eastern Zhou (771–256 BC). Traditional historiography also refers to the Spring and Autumn period (770–476 BC) and the Warring States period (475–221 BC). With the advent of the Zhou, China gradually entered a feudal stage, a description that Jacques Gernet not unreasonably rejects but which is used quite willingly by contemporary Chinese historians to characterise Chinese society from the Western Zhou to modern times.[2] While not entering this particular debate here, it is worthwhile to emphasise that the original meaning of the term *fengjian*, usually translated as 'feudal' or 'feudalism', is 'to grant a fief', a practice that was instituted precisely during the Zhou dynasty. This system, Jacques Gernet notes, 'which made it possible to grant to an aristocratic family a power both religious and military over a precisely defined domain . . . was in the last analysis only a replica of royalty within a vast hierarchy of families and domains'.[3] It was in this way that fiefdoms were formed, and their increasing power was to culminate in the undermining of royal authority.

Medical practice during the Western Zhou witnessed the beginnings of an organisation. The term *yi* (physician) already referred at this time to differing functions, to the extent that one might even speak of specialisation. At the top of the medical hierarchy were the *yishi* (master physicians), although according to the Rites of Zhou (*Zhouli*) there were several categories of physician at court, each one responsible for a particular function. There were, for example, *jiyi* (physicians for the cure of illness), who were concerned with internal medicine, while it was the function of the *yangyi* (physicians for the treatment of wounds) to treat cutaneous affections, injuries, traumatisms and fractures. Finally, there were *shiyi* (physicians for nutrition), who acted as dieticians. There also existed 'physicians for animals', the first Chinese veterinarians. These medical practitioners based their diagnoses on the theory of *yin* and *yang* (to be discussed more fully later) which, at the time, observes Ming Wong,

> was applied to the patient's environment, that is to say to the elements that surrounded the patient. Heaven was *yang*, while earth was *yin*. Man had to adapt to the internal as well as the external world, and was subject to the influence of water (in winter), fire (in summer), wood (in spring),[4] metal (in autumn) and finally to that of the earth.

Ming Wong also mentions the 'five elements' (wood, fire, earth, metal, water), but again will be discussed more fully when introducing *Huangdi Neijing* (Yellow Emperor's *Classic of Internal Medicine*), whose philosophy rested on these two theories conceived nearly 3,000 years ago.

The antiquity of the principles on which traditional Chinese medicine depended has been confirmed by the 1973 discovery in the number three tomb at Mawangdui[5] of medical tracts that probably antedate the *Huangdi Neijing*, the oldest Chinese work on medicine. The *Huangdi Neijing* has up until now been regarded as the first medical treatise to use the term *jingmai*, usually translated as 'meridian', the channel through which circulated vital energy. However, two of the works discovered at Mawangdui, *Zubi Shiyi Mai Jiujing* and *Yingyang Shiyi Mai Jiujing*, also refer to 'meridians', although they mention only eleven instead of the twelve cited by traditional Chinese medicine since the compilation of *Huangdi Neijing*. It is thought therefore that these three works represent three stages in the formation of the theory of *jingmai*, especially as the two works discovered at Mawangdui mention only the character *mai*.[6]

Another work discovered at Mawangdui, *Wushier Bingfang*, also testifies to the existence of medical and pharmaceutical knowledge in ancient China. With its 'fifty-two prescriptions against fifty-two ailments', it can claim to be one of the earliest Chinese pharmaceutical documents. Its proposed cures concern ailments whose treatment is primarily dependent on internal medicine, surgery, obstetrics, paediatrics and medicine for the 'five organs' (e.g. eyes, ears, mouth). The document also contains a description of a condition that in all likelihood resembles leprosy. Compared to the *Classic of Mountains and Seas (Shanhaijing)*, which merely notes that a certain plant can cure a particular illness, *Wushier Bingfang* represents an important step forward in the history of Chinese medicine. It lists, in fact, 242 drugs (*Shen'nong Bencaojing* lists 365) of mineral, plant and animal origin.

A number of medicinal plants likewise appear in the *Classic of Odes (Shijing)*, which Confucius described as having 'helped in the naming of birds, beasts, plants and trees'.[7] The *Classic of Odes*, the earliest anthology of Chinese poems, was compiled in the sixth century BC, although some of the poems date from the eleventh century BC. The anthology contains the names of fifty medicinal plants, among which is the kudzu vine (*Pueraria lobata*):

> The kudzu vine stretches long into the distance
> Right up to the centre of the valley,
> and its leaves are bountiful.
> The orioles hover and gather among the bushes,
> which echo to the sound of their song.

This creeping plant (*ge* in Chinese) is a generous source of textile fibre:

> The plant is cut and boiled
> To enable one to weave delicate and coarse cloth,
> Which one never gets tired in wearing.[8]

The author of this early poem, however, says nothing of the plant's edible possibilities nor of its therapeutic value. Today it grows wild throughout China, with the exception of Tibet and Xinjiang. Traditional Chinese medicine employs it especially in the treatment of influenza, acute gastritis and enteritis, infant diarrhoea and dysentery.[9] Included among the other plants mentioned in the *Classic of Odes* are the madder-wort (*Rubia cordifolia*), artemisia and various fruit trees such as those of the jujube, pear, peach and the plum, whose seeds and flesh are used in traditional medicine.

Moreover, a growing interest in alchemy during Zhou times foreshadowed a medical chemistry. By alchemy is meant the preparation of elixirs designed to prolong human life. Joseph Needham observes that 'early chemistry in China was, right from the start, really alchemy since it alone was preoccupied with the search for immortality'.[10] Needham, the historian of Chinese science and technology, also notes the absence of any prejudice against the use of mineral drugs and sees this as one of the origins of the alchemical tradition in ancient China. Finally, a reading of the *Rites of Zhou* (*Zhouli*) reveals that at the beginning of the first millennium before Christ people in China were preoccupied with nutritional and even sexual hygiene.

The Hundred Schools of Thought

In the words of Henri Maspero and Etienne Balazs, the Western Zhou was doomed to disappear quickly. In their book *History and Institutions of Ancient China*, they write: 'The development of the country as a whole, the growth of population and the prosperity of the feudal states inevitably exacerbated the decline of central control while also highlighting differences, and hence friction, among the feudal states themselves'.[11] The Spring and Autumn period experienced the competition and conflict that anticipated the Warring States period, a time when seven principal states engaged in interminable wars during the fourth and third centuries BC in order to achieve hegemony. These 'warring states' progressively absorbed their smaller neighbours. This 'constant war-fever', in Jacques Gernet's words, lasted until 221 BC, when the ruler of Qin succeeded in defeating his rivals and unifying China.

This time of crisis and dramatic change threw up a number of significant personalities, first among whom was Confucius, making this period one of the most outstanding in the history of Chinese thought. Confucius (551–479 BC) described the superior man (*junzi*) as one who 'preached only what he practised'. The superior man strove to realise *ren*, a central concept in Confucius's thought although he never fully defined it, simply replying to one of his disciples that *ren* was 'to love others'. Confucianism can be seen in terms of an 'active' humanism, to be utilised especially by the ruler: 'Choose yourself to abide by the moral way and the people will improve'.[12] This political concern was shared by Laozi, the founder of Daoism, who may have lived during the sixth century BC. Laozi, the presumed author of *Daodejing* (*Classic of the Way and of Virtue*), called on feudal rulers and kings to observe the *dao*, and by so doing 'everyone would, of themselves, be transformed'.[13]

Confucianism, which was enthusiastically embraced by Mencius (c. 372–289 BC) and added to by Xun Zi (c. 298–238 BC), aroused not only the opposition of the Daoists – the *Zhuangzi*, attributed to Zhuang Zhou (c. 328–295 BC), for example, takes issue on numerous occasions with Confucius's ideas – but also that of the Legalists and Mohists. The most important representatives of

Legalism, a political philosophy concerned with power that held sway during the third and fourth centuries BC, were Shang Yang (c. 390–338 BC) and Han Fei (280–233 BC). The thought of Mo Di (c. 480–400 BC), founder of the Mohist school, was influential until the third century BC, although the *Zhuangzi* regretted that 'it fell far short of the ideal doctrines of the ancient kings'.[14] Amid the competing voices of the 'hundred schools of thought' could also be heard the sophists such as Gongsun Long (c. 325–250 BC), who unsettled other thinkers with such celebrated paradoxes as 'a white horse is not a horse'. Finally, there was the poetic melancholy of Qu Yuan (c. 353–284 BC):

> I sigh deeply and shed tears,
> Grieving in the wake of the people's suffering . . .
> The age is so troubled and disorder grows,
> How can I tarry here much longer? .
> The orchid and the iris no longer exude their scent . . .[15]

The influence of Confucianism, Daoism, Legalism and other schools of thought such as that of the *yin* and the *yang* was significant for the development of medicine at this time, providing medical practice with its theoretical foundations. Such influence is clearly evident in the *Huangdi Neijing*, whose philosophy rests on key concepts that have since governed traditional Chinese medicine: *qi*, *yin* and *yang*, and *wu xing*.

The concept of *qi*, which can be variously translated as 'air', 'vapour' or 'breath', occupies an important place in Chinese philosophy. Mencius, for example, endowed the concept with a moral dimension, while Xun Zi saw it as the source of the cosmos. This latter notion is elaborated upon by the *Huangdi Neijing*, which refers to *qi* as one of the components of the human body. As used in traditional Chinese medicine, the term is usually translated as 'breath' or 'energy'. Pierre Carrère observes that 'essentially *qi* appears to be associated with the energy that ensures the cohesion of atoms making up all matter'.[16] In animating matter, *qi* controls the working of the organs through which it circulates. Any lack or stagnation of this 'vital' energy engenders problems. A headache, constipation, fever, abdominal pain, arthralgia or dyspnoea can result from a weakening of *qi*. Likewise, the blocking of *qi* can produce ailments as diverse as lumbago, dysmenorrhoea, dysphagia and even the appearance of a tumour.

The origin of the concepts of *yin* and *yang* is lost in the mists of Chinese history. During the eighth century BC, according to the *Guoyu* (*Discourses of the States*), a historical work dating from the

Spring and Autumn period, a certain Bo Yangfu referred to *yin* and *yang* in explaining the phenomenon of earthquakes. *Yin* was identified with the earth, the moon, darkness, everything feminine, coldness and passivity. *Yang* was identified with heaven, the sun, light, everything masculine, warmth and energy. *Yin* and *yang* also represent the broken and unbroken lines of the *Book of Changes* (*Yijing*), a work of divination possibly compiled during the Western Zhou. The *Book of Changes* comprises a set of eight trigrams (representing all combinations of unbroken and broken lines) which are then paired to form sixty-four hexagrams. The most harmonious of the combinations unite the two elements of *yin* and *yang*, which are seen as inseparable, each one dependent on the other. Lao Zi observed:

> The *dao* gives rise to one,
> One gives rise to two,
> Two give rise to three,
> And three give rise to the ten thousand beings.
> The ten thousand beings all carry *yin* on their shoulders
> And embrace *yang* in their arms . . .

This idea of the coexistence of *yin* and *yang* within each being pervades traditional Chinese medicine. In the *Huangdi Neijing*, Qi Bo, physician to the Yellow Emperor, says that the *yin* and *yang* are 'the source of the ten thousand beings'. Good health depends on the equilibrium of these two elements, while an excess of one or the other provokes illness. The *Zouzhuan* (*Commentary of Zuo*), a chronicle of the Zhou period, attributes to Yi He (who lived around 540 BC), a noted physician from the state of Qin, the following words:

> The six influences are *yin, yang,* the wind, rain, darkness and light . . . an excess of *yin* causes chills; an excess of *yang* causes fever; an excess of wind causes ailments of the limbs; an excess of rain causes ailments of the stomach; an excess of darkness affects the mind; an excess of light affects the feelings.

The theory of the five elements or phases (*wuxing*) has a history of nearly 3,000 years. Drawing on the *Hongfan*, a tract dating from the Zhou period, the *Huangdi Neijing* describes the five elements thus: 'Heaven has four seasons and five elements to allow cultivation, growth, harvesting and storing. It produces cold, heat, drought, humidity and wind. Man has five vital organs that transform the five influences to engender happiness, anger, vexation, sadness and fear.' The five elements – wood, fire, earth, metal and water – rep-

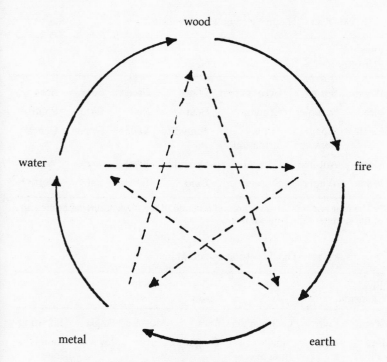

FIGURE 2.1   From *Zhongyixue Jichu* (Beijing: Renmin Weisheng Chubanshe, 1984).

resent forces (the Chinese word, *xing*, implies 'to proceed', 'to do', 'to act') that react against each other. Wood brings forth fire, fire produces ashes (that is soil or earth), earth brings forth metal, metal produces steam when heated (water), and water produces trees (wood). On the other hand, earth is broken by wood, water is contained by earth, fire is extinguished by water, metal is melted by fire, and wood is shaped by metal. Figure 2.1 above illustrates these reactions:

The five elements are linked to nature and man through a whole series of connections. Thus wood corresponds to spring, germination and wind, as well as to the liver, gall-bladder and mouth, and to anger. From a reading of the *Huangdi Neijing*, which contains such passages as 'The east gives rise to wind, wind produces wood, wood gives birth to acid, acid nourishes the liver, the liver supports the muscles, and the muscles sustain the heart', a chart (Tables 2.1 and 2.2 below) showing the most essential links can be drawn up:

TABLE 2.1   The five elements and Nature.

Five Elements			Nature			
Wood	Spring	Germination	Wind	Green	Sour	East
Fire	Summer	Growth	Heat	Red	Bitter	South
Earth	'Long* Summer'	Trans- formation	Humidity	Yellow	Sweet	Centre
Metal	Autumn	Harvest	Drought	White	Acrid	West
Water	Winter	Storage	Cold	Black	Salty	North

* The four seasons 'revolve' around a period of ten days occurring at the end of the summer: 'the long summer'.

TABLE 2.2   The five elements and Man.

Five Elements			Man			
Wood	Liver	Gall-bladder	Eyes	Muscles	Anger	Shouting
Fire	Heart	Small Intestine	Tongue	Ducts	Joy	Laugh- ing
Earth	Spleen	Stomach	Mouth	Flesh	Sadness	Singing
Metal	Lungs	Large Intestine	Nose	Skin and Hair	Vexation	Wailing
Water	Kidneys	Bladder	Ears	Bones	Fear	Groan- ing

Between the eighth and third centuries BC, the theoretical bases of Chinese medicine as outlined above were formulated. The *Huangdi Neijing* was the culmination of this long process. At the same time, principles of hygiene and preventive medicine became commonplace. This can be seen from the practices described in texts as diverse as the *Book of Changes*, *Classic of Odes*, *Zuozhuan* and even the *Guoyu*.[17] The *Classic of Odes*, for example, refers to the use of ice for conserving food:

> In the twelfth month, the ice is broken. Crack! Crack!
> And in the first month it is stored in the ice-cave.[18]

According to the *Book of Changes*, the appropriate behaviour of the superior man is not only 'to take care with one's words' but also to 'be moderate in eating and drinking'. With such advice in mind, the *Analects* (*Lunyu*) of Confucius describes the dietary habits of the wise man:

> It is permissible to eat polished rice and finely-minced meat. One does not eat sour rice or meat and fish that has spoiled. One does not eat food that has gone off colour or has a bad smell, is not prepared properly or in season, is not properly cut up or served with appropriate seasoning. Even if meat were abundant, one must not eat more meat than rice. Only wine is not limited, but one must never abuse it. Wine and dried meat bought from a shop are to be avoided. Even with ginger still on the table, one must never eat more than is proper.[19]

Special attention was paid to avoiding contaminated water. The *Book of Changes* notes that 'Muddied water from the well is not drunk' and adds that 'only clear and fresh water from the well is drunk'. The *Lushi Chunqiu* (*Spring and Autumn Annals of Master Lu*) describes the effects of drinking water according to its quality. Thus 'where the water is airy or light, baldness and goitre will be commonplace; where the water is heavy, there will be lameness . . .'. Anthrax and acne will break out 'where the water is tart', but 'where the water is mild there will be many fine complexions'. The growth of towns during the fourth and third centuries BC brought in their wake significant changes in daily life, one of which involved the construction of sewers. Archaeological evidence testifies to their existence in urban areas from the Warring States period onwards.

Yellow Emperor's Classic of Internal Medicine (Huangdi Neijing)

The *Huangdi Neijing* comprises two parts: Plain Questions (*Suwen*) and Efficacious Pivot (*Lingshu*). The earliest reference to the work occurs in the *Hanshu* (*History of the Han Dynasty*) compiled by Ban Gu (AD 32–92), where it is listed as one of the seven 'classics of medicine' (*yijing*). The questions posed by the Yellow Emperor and his advisers concern not just medicine but also philosophy, astronomy, meteorological phenomena, geography and biology. The work thus brings together various branches of scientific knowledge known to exist in early China. The *Huangdi Neijing* is the product of a group of different authors, demonstrated by the repetitions and contradictions within the text, as well as by the differences in style. Compiled sometime during the Warring States period, it probably began as scattered tracts that were later collected in one book and given a title. It was then finally added to, rearranged, and revised. It seems likely that the *Huangdi Neijing* did not take on its final shape and content until the Western Han dynasty (206 BC to AD 25). It is significant, for example, that Sima Qian (145–86 BC), the greatest of Chinese historians, makes no mention of the *Huangdi Neijing* in his *Shiji* (*Records of the Grand Historian*).

One wonders why both the title and content of the work refer to the Yellow Emperor. This legendary monarch was much venerated, particularly among Daoist thinkers and those of the *yin* and *yang* school. Significantly, the influence of these two strands of thought pervades the *Huangdi Neijing*. The very name of the Yellow Emperor, like that of Shen'nong for the *Shen'nong Bencaojing*, thus anticipates the content of the work. Reference to the *Suwen*, one of the two sections of the *Huangdi Neijing*, is first made by Zhang Ji, a physician of the second century BC, although he makes no mention of *Neijing* (*Classic of Internal Medicine*). We know, however, that Zhang Ji was referring to the *Huangdi Neijing*, since this is specifically mentioned by Huangfu Mi (third century AD) in his treatise on acupuncture. The *Lingshu*, on the other hand, is not mentioned in the *History of the Han Dynasty*, neither is it specifically referred to by Zhang Ji and Huangfu Mi. However, Huangfu Mi refers to a work entitled *Zhenjing* (*Classic of Acupuncture*), which Zhang Ji simply refers to as *The Nine Volumes*. This work, in fact, is none other than the *Lingshu*.[20]

The *Lingshu*, or *Zhenjing* (*zhen* means 'needle'), is more concerned with acupuncture, while the *Suwen* deals with 'essential questions' pertaining to anatomy, physiology and therapy in the form of dialogues between the Yellow Emperor and his advisers, particularly Qi Bo. According to these dialogues, man has five *zang* organs – liver, heart, spleen, lungs and kidneys – which correspond to the principle of *yin*, and another six organs, known as *fu*, which correspond to the principle of *yang*. These latter comprise the gall-bladder, stomach, large intestine, small intestine, urinary bladder and the 'triple burner'. The 'triple burner' does not refer to a real organ but describes the digestive, cardiorespiratory and urinary functions. Energy (*qi*) circulates within the body through a network of twelve channels, or meridians (*jingmai*), which are compared in chapter 27 of the *Suwen* to waterways:

> Heaven is covered with the constellations, earth with water-ways, man with channels. When heaven and earth are temperate, the waters are calm; when heaven is cold and earth frozen, the waters stagnate; when heaven is warm and the

earth scorched, the waters boil; when the wind blows violently, the waters break into waves.

According to chapter 62 of the *Suwen*, devoted to the regulation of the channels, illness originates with a state of either depletion (*xu*) or repletion (*shi*). Invigorating action is recommended for the former and dispelling action for the latter. The *Lingshu* applies this principle to acupuncture, where the use of needles is sometimes to invigorate and replenish and sometimes to disperse blockages. The condition of scarcity or excess is interpreted by an examination of the pulse, of which there are nine reference points (*hou*). As Qi Bo explains to the Yellow Emperor, 'Man has three parts, each one possessing three sets of pulse by which one might ascertain the chances of survival, control the hundred illnesses, and harmonise the states of depletion and excess . . .'. J. Borsarello notes that the condition of a particular organ can be ascertained through an examination of the pulse, which reveals the palpitation of the relevant artery. Thus 'diagnosis of the wrist pulse, which is connected to the radial artery, provides information on the crucial cardiac, hepatic and intestinal functions'.[21]

Only a brief description has been given here of the content of the *Huangdi Neijing*, and there will be need to return again to the 'bible' of Chinese medicine which, for example, attributes to the heart the function of controlling blood circulation and to the brain the function of controlling the medulla (marrow). It should also be noted that in the case of therapy, the *Huangdi Neijing* recommends acupuncture, moxibustion, massage and drugs, as well as hydrotherapy, according to the particular circumstances. It also offers nutritional advice:

> If one eats food that is too salty, this leads to coagulation of the blood vessels and changes one's complexion; if one eats food that is too bitter, the skin dries up and one's skin hairs fall out; if one eats food that is too sharp, the muscles contract and one's nails wither; if one eats food that is too acrid, the flesh shrinks and one's lips swell up; if one eats food that is too bland, the bones ache and cause the hair to drop out . . .

Qin Yueren, a Popular Hero in Early Chinese Medicine

Qin Yueren (c. 407–310 BC), better known under the name Bian Que, has become a legendary 'miracle-doctor' said to be capable of exchanging the hearts of two patients. The *Liezi* records that he 'gave each of the patients strong wine that put them to sleep for three days. He then made incisions into their chests, examined their hearts, and replaced them in the other patient's body. After drinking

some magical liquor, they regained consciousness.'[22] The more
realistic Han Fei, well-known Legalist of the third century BC, gives
a more historically accurate picture of Qin Yueren, who has become
the Chinese equivalent of Aesculapius, Roman god of Medicine:

> On visiting King Huan of Cai, Bian Que remarked: 'Your
> lordship is ill. For the moment, only the surface of your body is
> affected, but if you fail to take precautions, the illness will
> become worse.' 'I'm not ill,' King Huan replied, whereupon
> Bian Que took his leave . . . Ten days later, Bian Que returned
> and remarked: 'Your lordship's illness has now affected the
> muscles. If you do not take precautions, it will become even
> worse.' King Huan would have nothing of this and Bian Que
> took his leave . . . Ten days later, he returned and observed:
> 'Your lordship's illness has now affected the intestines and
> stomach. If you continue to refuse taking action, the illness will
> become still worse. Again King Huan brushed the advice aside,
> and Bian Que took his leave . . . Ten days later, King Huan
> noticed Bian Que turn away from his presence. The king sent a
> servant to enquire of Bian Que why he had turned away. Bian
> Que answered: 'When an illness affects the surface of the body,
> a lotion or a hot compress can cure it; when an illness affects
> the muscles, the use of needles can cure it; when an illness
> affects the intestines and stomach, decoctions can cure it; but
> when an illness affects the bones there is nothing else to do but
> leave things to fate. Since the king's illness has now in fact
> affected the bones, I saw no reason to recommend that he take
> care of himself.' Five days later, King Huan, racked with illness
> throughout his body, had Bian Que searched for, but he had
> already departed for the state of Qin. King Huan died soon
> afterwards.[23]

The *Shiji* (*Records of the Grand Historian*) details Qin Yueren's
biography. A young innkeeper of a town located in the present-day
province of Hebei, Qin Yueren was introduced to medicine by a
certain Chang Sangjun, who revealed to Qin his 'secret prescriptions'.
Qin Yueren then practised his medical skills throughout the states
of Zhao, Guo, Qi and Qin, accompanied on his travels by his
disciples Ziyang and Zibao. In this way, he had occasion to revive
the heir-apparent of Guo, assumed to be dead after a fainting fit left
him unconscious. Qin's growing reputation prompted King Huan of
Qi to invite Qin to his court. According to the *Shiji*, when Qin
Yueren examined the king he advised him to take care before the
illness became worse and gradually affected the blood-vessels,
intestines, stomach and, finally, the bones. Sima Qian's account

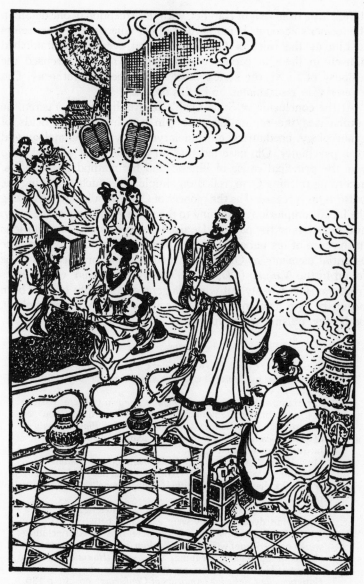

FIGURE 2.2   Qin Yueren revives the heir-apparent of Guo. From *Zhongguo Gudai Yixuejia De Gushi* (Shanghai: Shaonian Ertong Chubanshe, 1979).

differs little from that of Han Fei, with the exception of one detail: in the former's account, Huan is ruler of Qi, whereas the latter refers to him as the ruler of Cai. Qin Yueren eventually established himself in the Qin capital of Xianyang, where he aroused the jealousy of Li Xi, the state's most senior medical authority. Qin Yueren was assassinated on Li Xi's orders.

At the conclusion of Sima Qian's biography of Qin Yueren, he emphasises the reputation that Qin acquired in the fields of gynaecology, paediatrics, otorhinolaryngology, ophthalmology and even psychiatry. Qin asserted that an imbalance of *yin* and *yang* was the principal cause of illness, and his method of diagnosis, according to Sima Qian, relied on simple rules such as 'taking the pulse' (Qin is regarded as the pioneer of Chinese pulsing), 'observing the facial complexion', 'listening to the noise vibrations' of the body, and questioning the patient. He used decoctions and fomentations in the cure of his patients, as well as practising acupuncture. The essential elements of Qin Yueren's theory and practice are to be found in the *Nanjing* (*Classic of Difficult Problems*), which dates from the Han dynasty but which is generally thought to have been begun by Qin Yueren himself. The work deals with physiology, pathology, pulsing and acupuncture.

Notes

1. *Entretiens de Confucius* (*Analects of Confucius*), translated from the Chinese by Anne Cheng (Paris: Editions de Seuil, 1981), p 152.
2. For example, Fan Wenlan, *Zhongguo Tongshi* (*General History of China*) (Beijing: Renmin chubanshe, 1978). On the Zhou, see in particular Zhao Guangxian, *Zhoudai Shehui Bianxi* (*Analysis of Zhou Society*) (Beijing: Renmin chubanshe, 1980).
3. Jacques Gernet, op. cit., p 54.
4. Ming Wong, 'La Médecine Chinoise Antique', in *Histoire de la Médecine, de la Pharmacie, de l'Art Dentaire et de l'Art Vétérinaire* (Paris: Société française d'éditions professionnelles médicales et pharmaceutiques, 1977), p 73.
5. The archaeological site at Mawangdui is located near Changsha. Three Han dynasty tombs were excavated between 1972 and 1974. Among notable discoveries were rare books (including works on medicine) written on silk cloth.
6. He Jiejun and Zhang Weiming, *Mawangdui Hanmu* (*The Han Tombs of Mawangdui*) (Beijing: Wenwu chubanshe, 1982).
7. *Entretiens de Confucius* (*Analects of Confucius*), op. cit., p 136.
8. *Le Livre de Poèmes* (*The Book of Odes*), translated from the Chinese by Dominique Hoizey (Reims: Albédo, 1986).
9. The chemical, pharmacological and clinical study of the *Pueraria lobata* (kudzu vine) has shown that the isoflavanoid elements lower tension, reduce cardiac rhythm and increase cerebral and coronary circulation. Ethanolic extract from the root of the kudzu

vine is prescribed today in the case of hypertension, angina pectoris and migraine. See Fang Qicheng, 'Some current study and research approaches relating to the use of plants in traditional Chinese medicine', *Journal of Ethnopharmacology,* no 2 (1980), pp 57–63.

10. Joseph Needham, *The Grand Titration* (London: Allen and Unwin, 1969), pp 69–70.

11. Henri Maspero and Etienne Balazs, *Histoire et Institutions de la Chine Ancienne* (Paris: PUF, 1967), p 21.

12. An entire chapter of the *Analects* is devoted to the art of governing. See Anne Cheng, op. cit., pp 95–101. It contains the celebrated saying: 'Let the ruler act as a ruler, the minister as a minister, the father as a father, and the son as a son'.

13. Laozi, *Daodejing*, translated by Liou Kia-hway in *Philosophes Taoistes* (Paris: Gallimard, 1980), p 40.

14. *Zhuangzi*, translated by Liou Kia-hway in *Philosophes Taoistes,* op. cit., p 351.

15. Huang Shengfa, *Qu Yuan et le Li Sao* (Beijing: Foreign Language Press, 1985).

16. *Le Pao Tsien Fa ou Comment Conserver Jeunesse et Santé Grâce aux Vieilles Méthodes Chinoises.* Commentary and translation by Pierre Carrère (Paris: Aubier-Montagne, 1979), p 30.

17. See Pan Jinling, 'Materials related to preventive medicine of the pre-Spring-Autumn and Spring-Autumn periods', *Zhonghua Yishi Zazhi* (Chinese Journal of Medical History), 16:2 (April 1986).

18. An ice-cave dating from the Spring and Autumn period was discovered near Fengxiang in Shaanxi province. It could hold 190 cubic metres of ice. See 'Shaanxi Fengxiang Chunqiu Qinguo Lingyin yizhi fajue jianbao', *Wenwu*, no 3 (1978), pp 43–7.

19. *Entretiens de Confucius (Analects of Confucius)*, op. cit., p 83. Confucius was once offered a medical substance. He accepted it, but 'not knowing its properties,' he said, 'I am not going to take the risk of trying it'.

20. See Liu Changlin, *Neijing de Zhexue he Zhongyixue de Fangfa* (Beijing: Kexue Chubanshe, 1985), pp 8–31.

21. J. Borsarello, *L'Acupuncture et l'Occident* (Paris: Fayard, 1974), p 131.

22. See Benedykt Grynpas's translation of the *Liezi*, op. cit., p 489.

23. Author's translation from *Han Feizi Jishi* (Shanghai: Renmin Chubanshe, 1974).

3

From the First Emperor to the Fall of the Han Dynasty, 221 BC to AD 220

From the First Emperor to the Yellow Turbans

During the eighth century AD, the poet Li Bai described in memorable verse the gestures and deeds of the 'first emperor', who united China in 221 BC:

The Qin ruler's reach extends to the six directions.
A fierce overlord with the look of a tiger,
With his brandished sword he cleaves asunder
   the floating clouds.
Princes come one after the other to the west
To bow before him . . .[1]

Qin Shi Huangdi, not content to unify China through force of arms, proceeded to standardise the differing systems of currency, writing and weights and measures then in use throughout the Chinese world. The severe legalist policies pursued by the first emperor met with opposition from the nobility and scholars, who were dealt with harshly. In particular, Qin Shi Huangdi ordered the infamous 'burning of the books' in 213 BC (treatises on divination, agriculture and medicine were spared) and had 460 scholars put to death as a warning to others.

The Qin empire fell apart as a result of peasant insurrections, but the succeeding Han dynasty founded by Liu Bang in 206 BC initially relied on the legalist institutions which it took over from the Qin. Jacques Gernet notes that 'at the beginning of the dynasty most of the laws and regulations in force under the First Emperor were retained'.[2] The Han dynasty dominated China for more than four hundred years (206 BC to AD 220), with an interim period (AD 9–23) during which the usurper Wang Mang attempted to found a new dynasty, separating the Western from the Eastern Han.

The Western Han, in order to combat incursions by nomadic

tribes (*xiongnu*) from the northern steppes, carried out a policy of expansion in Mongolia and central Asia. The dynasty likewise extended its reach to Manchuria, Korea, South China and Vietnam. At home, the silk trade, the principal source of commercial wealth (it was during this period that the 'Silk Road' became a regular communication route), so enhanced the influence of merchants that the authorities felt compelled to intervene more in the economy. The state monopolies in iron and salt, in fact, gave rise to a vigorous debate in 81 BC, a summary of which has been preserved in a work entitled *Yantielun* (*Debate on Salt and Iron*).[3]

The last years of the Eastern Han in the second century AD experienced a widespread agrarian crisis which led to popular revolts inspired by Daoist and millenarian sects. A late Han text, the *Laozi Bianhuajing* (*Classic of Lao Zi's Transformations*), spoke of the hope of Lao Zi's messiah-like return:

> The people are afflicted, and ills are heaped to overflowing.
> Everywhere is famine.
> I will change destiny
> And overturn the rule of Han.[4]

The Yellow Turbans succeeded in undermining the dynasty in AD 184, leaving China in the hands of army generals. The most famous of these generals was Cao Cao, whose warlike plots and schemes initiated the Three Kingdoms period in the third century AD.

Danielle and Vadime Elisseeff observe that 'because of the works of art it encouraged, the Han period appears increasingly with the passage of time to have been an era of brilliance'.[5] The jade shrouds of Prince Liu Sheng and his consort, discovered at Mancheng in Hebei province, provide striking testimony to this. The Chinese genius also manifested itself at this time in the fields of science and technology, with Zhang Heng inventing the first seismograph in the second century AD. In the realm of philosophy, the thought of Wang Chong (AD 27–97) embodied a rational materialism. This was also a pioneering period for historiography, with Sima Qian's *Shiji* serving as a model for future dynastic histories such as the *Hanshu* (*History of the Han*), compiled by Ban Gu at the end of the first century AD. In religion, the Han period saw the influx of Buddhism, which initially appeared as a new Daoist sect. During the reign of Emperor Huan (AD 147–68), in fact, a double cult to Lao Zi and Buddha developed, although the latter seemed to many at the time none other than the reincarnated Lao Zi.

How to Acquire Immortality

Qin Shi Huangdi was haunted by the idea of death. According to
the *Shiji*, he sought the elixir of immortality and attempted to
communicate with the immortals. He sent the Daoist shaman Xu
Fu to seek out the immortals among the islands which they were
thought to inhabit:

> Xu Fu has been sent along with the daughters of Qin.
> Who can say when their ship will return . . .[6]

The same obsession apparently gripped Emperor Wu of the Han,
who came to the throne in 140 BC. The *Han Wudi Neizhuan*
(*Unofficial History of Han Wudi*), a Daoist tract probably dating
from the sixth century AD, recounts in story form the meeting
between Emperor Wu and the Queen Mother of the West
(*Xiwangmu*). She informs him of the existence of 100 drugs,
inaccessible to mortals, with such fantastic names as 'the essence of
the moon that provides 10,000 years of life', 'the eyeball of the
White Dragon' and the 'giant weed of the Milky Way'.[7]

Henri Maspero has emphasised in one of his essays on Chinese
religion that early Daoism was concerned above all else to acquaint
its followers with the secret of longevity (*changsheng*). Thus, during
the Han period, 'one had to seek to develop within oneself an
internal embryo gifted with immortality, which would take shape,
grow and then transform the mortal body into a refined and buoyant
immortal being, in the same way a cicada or a snake casts off its old
skin'.[8] The candidate for longevity, in addition to practising alchemy
and following dietary rules, had to combine gymnastic, respiratory
and sexual exercises. Virtuous conduct was also required, and this
was no doubt why the author of a hagiography dedicated to a
legendary Daoist sage had his hero perform good deeds before
receiving the instruction of an immortal. The Daoist sage was
advised to partake of a simple diet consisting of sesame, rhubarb or
the bark of a peach-tree, which were considered useful 'to prolong
the years and enhance longevity', although not being capable of
avoiding death.[9] We shall return later to the subject of alchemy
when discussing Ge Hong, an important Chinese alchemist of the
early fourth century AD, but it is significant that already in 133 BC a
certain Li Shaojun, according to the *Shiji*, connected gold with
longevity and even immortality.

> If one makes offerings to the stove-spirit, one can change
> natural substances. If one succeeds in changing natural
> substances, the cinnabar can be transformed into gold. When

this gold has been produced, it can be made into plates and dishes for eating and drinking. Whoever uses these plates and dishes can prolong their life.[10]

These various practices to prolong life will be further discussed later, but here it might be interesting to mention specifically a kind of gymnastic exercise known as *daoyin*. This exercise was certainly practised during the Spring and Autumn period, and is recommended by the *Huangdi Neijing* as well as by the two most celebrated physicians at the end of the Han, Zhang Zhongjing and Hua Tuo. Excavations at the number three tomb at Mawangdui have produced a painting on silk representing forty-four persons (men and women), either fully clothed or naked to the waist, who are executing the movements of this gymnastic exercise commended by therapists, but also recommended for Daoist followers seeking longevity. The *Zhuangzi* mentions that

> Whoever exhales and inhales, breathing vigorously and calmly, who expels stale air and imbibes fresh air, who suspends oneself like a bear and stretches out one's limbs like a bird, is seeking none other than longevity. Such is the ideal of those who cultivate their bodies by stretching and contracting (*daoyin*).[11]

'Suspending oneself like a bear' and 'stretching out like a bird' are precisely the kind of movements represented on the Mawangdui painting, which also depicts other positions borrowed from the animal world. Several inscriptions discovered at the Mawangdui tomb specify the therapeutic benefits of certain positions; for example a particular exercise is recommended to combat numbness, another to combat painful knees, or another even to combat deafness.[12]

How did the Marchioness of Dai Die?

Archaeologists who began to excavate the number one Han tomb at Mawangdui in 1972 unexpectedly discovered the well-preserved remains of a woman. She was the consort of Licang, marquis of Dai and chief minister of Changsha principality. The couple lived during the early years of the Western Han and the wife had outlived her husband, who died in 186 BC. The information gathered as a result of a post-mortem conducted on the woman's corpse (she was approximately fifty years of age at the moment of decease) has relevance for the study of anatomy, histology, pathology and biochemistry. The following details are drawn from a study published under the direction of the Hunan Institute of Medicine, and particular attention is paid to pathology.[13]

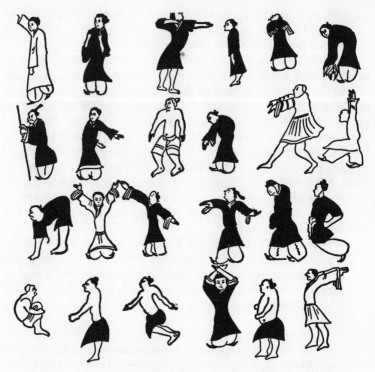

FIGURE 3.1   The *daoyin* gymnastic exercise. From a silk painting
excavated from the number three Han tomb at Mawangdui, in
Mawangdui Hanmu (Beijing: Wenwu Chubanshe, 1982).

Death apparently occurred shortly after the consumption of a
melon, numerous pips of which were discovered in the gullet,
stomach and intestines of the deceased. Analysis of physical changes
to the body and of the causes of death reveal that the Marchioness
of Dai suffered from disseminated sclerosis in the cavities of the
thoracic aorta, abdominal aorta and other arteries. Lesions to the
coronary arteries are even more in evidence, especially the left
coronary artery, whose cavity had been reduced by fifty to seventy-
five per cent or even more. The Marchioness had also been affected
by gallstones, the presence of which was noted in both the choledoch
and hepatic ducts. It would seem that schistosomiasis had been
another affliction, since schistosoma eggs covered in fibrous
connective tissue were found. Pathological deterioration was
discovered elsewhere, such as calcified tubercular nodules and a
badly-set fracture of the right radius and ulna. Moreover, a slipped

disc of the lumbar vertebra must have brought pain to the back and legs, forcing the Marchioness to support herself with a cane. This is, in fact, how she is represented on the funerary trappings that covered her tomb.

It is clear that the Marchioness of Dai died suddenly, most probably during an attack of biliary colic that provoked a coronary thrombosis. There is evidence that attempts were made to cure her, since medicinal plants were discovered among the funerary objects inside the tomb. These medicinal plants will be discussed when dealing with the *Classic of Herbal Medicine* (*Shen'nong Bencaojing*). Finally, it should be remembered that it was in the number three tomb at Mawangdui that the medical works discussed in the previous chapter (because they probably antedated the *Huangdi Neijing*) were discovered.

Liu Sheng, Brother of the Emperor

It is not known whether the Marchioness of Dai resorted to acupuncture; however, Liu Sheng, elder brother of Emperor Wu of the Han, who died in 113 BC, did make use of this therapeutic method. Needles were found in the tomb of this prince, whom history has described as a rather dissolute character. The needles, totalling nine in all, are made of gold (four) and silver (five) and are shaped differently according to specific function. The *Huangdi Neijing* distinguished nine kinds of needle, each one having a precise usage: the 'round' (*yuan*) served to massage the points (*xue*) on which to penetrate the skin with the aid, for example, of a 'bristle' (*hao*) needle, that is to say a needle 'as fine as a bristle-hair'. Among the nine needles discovered in Liu Sheng's tomb, four kinds have been definitively recognised, in particular the 'round' and 'bristle' needles. Also included was the 'pointed' (*feng*) needle, which was triangular in shape and used to induce bleeding.[14]

During the Han dynasty, two physicians were especially renowned in the practice of acupuncture and moxibustion, Fu Weng and Guo Yu. The name of Fu Weng, literally 'the old gentleman of the Fu', evokes the image of an elderly person (*weng*) fishing on the banks of the River Fu. If not for his reputation acquired by a widespread practice of acupuncture, very little would be known of Fu Weng, who lived during the first century AD. He wrote a treatise on acupuncture and pioneered a method for taking the pulse. Fu's disciple, Guo Yu, was officially employed at the court of Emperor He, whose reign began in AD 89. On one occasion, the emperor wondered why Guo Yu obtained better results among the ordinary people than among the privileged. Guo Yu listed four reasons why the latter had problems, of which 'love of idleness and dislike of work' was just as important in his view as 'not taking care with one's body'. One of the disciples of Hua Tuo, an important physician of the late Han, was also well versed in acupuncture. Known as Fan A, he extended its application to cover parts of the body hitherto deemed not possible, the back and the thorax.[15]

The *Shen'nong Bencaojing* (*Classic of Herbal Medicine*)

Political expansion and the growth of commercial relations during the Han introduced China to new plants such as the alfalfa and the vine from *xiyu* ('western countries'), that is regions situated to the west of the Dunhuang oasis on the silk route. It was also during this period that the walnut-tree made its appearance. Previously unknown medicinal plants from South China (such as the longan and litchi) added to the pharmacopoeia of which physicians made use to treat their patients. They were also able to utilise other ingredients in the composition of medicines, such as the horn of the rhinoceros, gland secretions of the musk-deer, and yellow amber.

Medicinal plants found in the number one tomb at Mawangdui illustrate the development of Chinese phytotherapy towards the beginning of the Christian era. In addition to the rhizomes of the *gaoliangjiang* (*Alpina officinarum*), the Marchioness of Dai's 'pharmaceutical cabinet' contained rhizomes of *maoxiang*, a gramineous plant known as *Hierochloë odorata*, strips of bark from the *Cinnamomum chekiangense*, seeds of *Zanthoxylum armatum*, flower-buds of the *Magnolia denudata*, rhizomes of *gaoben* (*Ligusticum jeholense*) and of the *Zingibar officinale* (the well-known ginger), roots of the asarum (*Asarum fargesii*) and flowers and achenes of the eupatorium.[16] It is very likely that the Marchioness of Dai was treated with these medicinal plants, some of which are mentioned in the *Huangdi Neijing*, such as the *gui*, a generic name for several kinds of lauraceae. These included cinnamon (*Cinnamomum cassia*), known as *mugui* or *rougui* in Chinese. Cinnamon is also mentioned in the *Shen'nong Bencaojing*, as well as *gaoben*, ginger, and hemp-agrimony.

The *Shen'nong Bencaojing* (*Classic of Herbal Medicine*) was compiled during the Han dynasty, probably sometime in the first century AD. It introduced a new term, *bencao* (literally 'essential herb'), and listed 365 drugs (*yao*, meaning 'medicinal herb' or 'remedy') of plant (252), animal (67) and mineral (46) origin. These drugs are classified as superior, average and inferior. The superior drugs, totalling 120, were known to be non-toxic and to produce an invigorating effect. According to the *Shen'nong Bencaojing*, such drugs helped prevent senescence, the most celebrated one being ginseng (*renshen*). The 120 average drugs, toxic in some cases, were used as a tonic to resist illness. Included in this category were the Chinese angelica and, notably, the ephedra (*mahuang*), which has been part of the Chinese pharmaceutical tradition for more than 2,000 years. The 125 inferior drugs, many of which are toxic (*du*, meaning 'poison'), are assigned an essentially therapeutic role by the *Shen'nong Bencaojing*. One example is the croton.

Besides ginseng (*Panax ginseng*), the angelica (*Angelica sinensis*), the ephedra (*Ephedra sinica*) and the croton (*Croton tiglium*), numerous other medicinal plants mentioned in the *Shen'nong Bencaojing* are still used today. Examples include sage (*Salvia miltiorrhiza*), asparagus (*Asparagus cochinchinensis*) the magnolia (*Magnolia liliflora*), the *Eucommia ulmoides*, the 'fruit with five flavours' (*Schisandra chinensis*), liquorice (*Glycyrrhiza uralensis*), the lily (*Lilium brownii*), the peony (*Paeonia suffruticosa*), rhubarb (*Rheum officinale*), kernel-seed of the peach (*Prunus persica*), kernel-seed of the Japanese plum (*Prunus japonica*), the euphorbia (*Euphorbia kansui*), Japanese dock (*Rumex japonicus*), the fritillary (*Fritillaria cirrhosa*), the *Achyranthes bidentata*, the *Anemarrhena asphodeloides*, the sweet-rush (*Acorus gramineus, Acorus calamus*), and 'heavenly flower powder' (*tianhuafen*), a common term for a kind of cucurbitaceous plant, *Trichosanthes kirilowii*.[17] The bezoar of an ox is mentioned as a drug of animal substance.

The properties of each drug are described. Ginseng, for example, is said to 'invigorate the five organs (*zang*) and calm the mind . . .', as well as 'to prolong life'. The place where each medicinal plant grows is also given in the *Shen'nong Bencaojing*; croton, for example, grows by the riverbank, while the 'fruit of five flavours' is to be found on the mountain-slope. The preparation of such medicinal plants is also concisely described; some need to be dried in the sun, others in the shade or over a fire. The discovery in Liu Sheng's tomb of a basin apparently to rinse such plants testifies to the care taken at that time to prepare drugs. Catherine Despeux, who has translated Zhang Zhongjing's *Shanghanlun*, a work of the second century AD that gives information on how some of the remedies during the Han were prepared,[18] notes that 'after an initial rinse and wash, the substance was either shredded or reduced to powder and then dried before being heated or soaked'. The *Shanghanlun*, an anthology of medical prescriptions discussed below, is similar to the *Wushier Bingfang* (*The Fifty-Two Prescriptions*), a medical text discovered at Mawangdui.

Another document that pertains to the history of Chinese medicine deserves mention: the ninety-two wooden tablets discovered in 1973 in a Han tomb at Wuwei (Gansu province). The thirty-odd deciphered medical prescriptions written on the tablets mention the names of 100 drugs, among which are sixty medicinal plants. These include the angelica, rhubarb, ephedra, ginseng, croton and ginger, as well as other plants mentioned in the *Shen'nong Bencaojing*, such as *Scutellaria baicalensis* and *Sophora flavencens*. The remedies are prescribed in the form of decoctions, pills, ointment, powder or medicinal alcohol. The excipient used in the preparation of these medicines is also mentioned: honey, pork grease and milk.[19]

The Medical Dossiers of Chunyu Yi

Chunyu Yi (215–167 BC?) was a native of Linzi, a town situated in present-day Shandong province. According to the *Shiji*, he was fascinated by medicine from childhood. As the organiser of a public granary, he was given the name Cang Gong ('Master of the Granary').

The twenty-five clinical observations made by Chunyu Yi and recounted in the *Shiji* are a mine of information on medical practice in early China. Moreover, Chunyu Yi was the first Chinese physician to keep 'medical records' on his patients. Each of his twenty-five observations is accompanied by the name of the patient, the name and nature of the illness, its cause, the treatment followed, the remedy used and the progress of the illness.

An official from the state of Qi came to Chunyi Yi with a decayed tooth. Chunyi Yi applied a moxa and then prescribed a decoction of *kushen* (*Sophora flavescens*). After several days, the pain was gone. Chunyi Yi based his diagnoses essentially on taking the pulse. It was by means of this that he examined a person from Qi by the name of Poshi and was able to ascertain a fatal lesion of the lungs, predicting imminent death from blackwater fever. Chunyi Yi treated his patients principally with drugs, usually in the form of decoctions, but he also made use of pills.

Zhang Zhongjing, the 'Sage of Medicine'

Zhang Zhongjing (AD 150–219?), also known as Zhang Ji, was born in Nanyang district, Henan province. Very little of his life is known besides hagiographical anecdotes from various sources, which simply confirm Zhang's established reputation as the 'sage of medicine'. The most famous episode concerning Zhang Zhongjing is his meeting with Wang Zhongxuan, to whom he remarked: 'It is clear you are ill. One day your eyebrows will drop out, and six months after that you will die. You need to take a decoction of the five minerals in order to avoid such a fate.' Wang Zhongxuan did not believe him. Shortly afterwards, noticing from Wang's complexion that he had not taken any precautionary measures, Zhang again urged his friend to follow his advice. Wang finally died, most probably from leprosy.

It was Zhang Bozu, a childhood friend, who introduced Zhang to medicine and encouraged him to follow a medical career at a time when China was sinking into chaos. The break-up of the Han empire and the resulting popular rebellions and their repression brought in their wake an increase in the number of epidemics. According to Zhang Zhongjing himself, more than two-thirds of the Zhang lineage (comprising approximately 200 members) died during the ten years after AD 196. Seven out of every ten who died succumbed to illnesses that Chinese traditional medicine groups under the generic name of *shanghan*. The term embraces various ailments caused by an external agent, from a simple chill to gastritis or cholera.[20] It was this situation that prompted Zhang to write *Shanghanlun* (*On Cold-induced Maladies*), based on his own experiences and building on the foundations laid by the *Huangdi Neijing* and *Nanjing*. He wrote several other works such as *Jingui Yaolue* (*Summary from the Golden Chest*).

The original manuscript of *Shanghanlun* is lost, but in the third century AD Wang Shuhe rewrote the essential content. There are many editions and commentaries on this important classic, which, in the words of Ming Wong, 'encompasses the general features of Chinese traditional medicine'.[21] The work is divided into six parts, each one corresponding to the six pairs of meridians or channels (*jing*): *taiyang, yangming, shaoyang, taiyin, shaoyin* and *jueyin*. The section dealing with illnesses of *taiyang* is the most elaborate. Such illnesses are manifested by headaches, stiffness of the neck and susceptibility to cold. Zhang Zhongjing further distinguished two kinds of ailment associated with the *taiyang* meridian: one he called *zhongfeng*, which was accompanied by fever and sweating, the other he called *shanghan*, which might or might not be accompanied by fever but which caused lumbago and vomiting.

Concerning treatment, Zhang recommended a decoction of *Cinnamomum cassia* when the patient 'shivers with fever, breathes heavily and feels nauseous'.[22] In the event of no improvement, Zhang offered several other solutions, depending on the patient's symptoms. If, after having taken the decoction of *Cinnamomum cassia*, the patient 'sweats profusely, feels uncomfortable, is thirsty and is still not cured, and if his pulse is high, then it is appropriate to take a decoction of "white tiger" and more ginseng'.[23] A decoction of *Pueraria lobata* is recommended if the patient 'has stiff back and muscles, does not breathe easily, and is susceptible to wind', while a decoction of *Ephedra sinica* is recommended if the patient 'is feverish, suffers from headache and backache, has painful loins and joints, is susceptible to the wind, and has dyspnoea'.[24] This phytotherapy is supplemented by dietary advice (no uncooked or cold food, or alcoholic drink) and by other therapeutic measures such as acupuncture and moxibustion.

Catherine Despeux justly points out that the renown of the *Shanghanlun* has less to do with its remedies than with 'its approach to each individual pathological case'. Thus, to cure an ailment associated with the *shaoyin* meridian, which manifests itself especially by 'a desire to vomit but being unable to do so', a peevish mood, a permanent state of drowsiness, diarrhoea and clear urine, the *Shanghanlun* prescribes principally a decoction of *Aconitum carmichaeli* 'if the patient has body-aches, the tips of his limbs are cold, and he has a painful back and joints'. On the other hand, a decoction of peach-blossom is prescribed 'if the patient has diarrhoea and purulent blood in the stool' and one of liquorice 'if the patient has a sore throat'.[25] The *Shanghanlun* might advise against the use of a particular decoction, and even against a purging. If there is a therapeutic error, the *Shanghanlun* notes that 'it is necessary to ascertain which error has been committed and to carry out new treatment in accordance with the appropriate method'.[26]

Hua Tuo, the Pioneer of Chinese Surgery

Hua Tuo (AD 141–208) was a native of Anhui province.[27] According to the *Houhanshu* (*History of the Later Han*), written in the fifth century AD, Hua Tuo went to study in Xuzhou (Jiangsu province). He turned down offers from various eminent persons to take up an official career, choosing medicine instead – a vocation to which he dedicated his entire life. During the course of his travels in the provinces of Jiangsu, Shandong, Anhui and Henan, he cured people along the way and gained much practical knowledge, never hesitating to learn from popular medical traditions. Apparently, his dealings with more important contemporaries were not so amicable. One such person was Cao Cao, ruler of northern China at the beginning of the third century, whom Hua Tuo treated for migraine. Hua Tuo, however, refused to enter his personal service; Cao Cao, out of spite, had him killed. Whatever the authenticity of this episode, Hua Tuo's renown has survived to the present. Numerous anecdotes concerning this important figure of early Chinese medicine

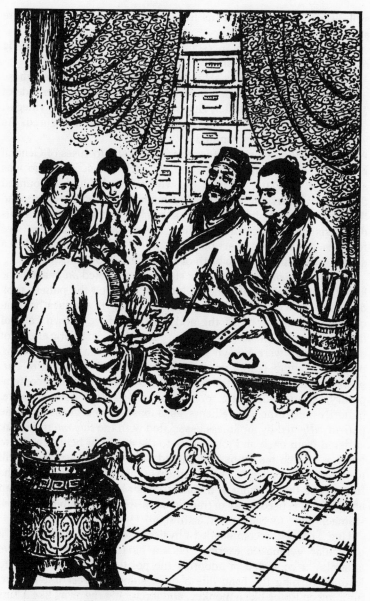

FIGURE 3.2   Zhang Zhongjing. From *Zhongguo Gudai Yixuejia De Gushi* (Shanghai: Shaonian Ertong Chubanshe, 1979).

still circulate today, while his life has been recounted in cartoon-strip.[28]

Some aspects of his personality and quick wit are briefly recounted in the *Houhanshu*:

> On the road one day, Hua Tuo met an ailing person whose pharynx was blocked. Hua Tuo advised: 'On the other side of the road is a cake-seller. Buy some crushed garlic and vinegar, drink three measures of the mixture and you will be cured.' As expected, the man vomited . . .

Another well-known anecdote concerns the twin foetuses of General Li's wife, who was suffering from stomach pains. Hua Tuo was asked to investigate. He took the woman's pulse and announced that she was carrying a foetus. The husband, taken aback, replied that his wife had already given birth. Hua Tuo persevered in his diagnosis since, according to him, there had in fact been two foetuses. He performed acupuncture on the patient and gave her a decoction to stimulate the birth of the second baby.

The *Houhanshu* recounts that Hua Tuo perfected an anaesthetic known as *mafeisan* (*san* means 'powder'), which the patient took dissolved in a fermented beverage. He used this anaesthetic in carrying out incisions of the abdomen, the first known case of laparotomy in the history of Chinese surgery. The narcotic effects of certain plants were known some time before Hua Tuo's time, in particular hemp (*Cannabis sativa*) and aconite (*Aconitum carmichaeli*), mentioned in the *Shen'nong Bencaojing*. Hua's contemporary, Zhang Zhongjing, prescribed a decoction using aconite, liquorice and other ingredients as a base in the event that the patient, affected by an illness associated with the *taiyang* meridian, suffered from back and joint pains to the extent of being unable to bend or stretch his limbs.[29] It should be noted that aconite is still used today in the treatment of arthritis. Hua Tuo is considered the first to use the blossom of a solanaceous plant (*mantuoluo*) as an analgesic. It is used today in traditional medicine to soothe tracheitis, stomach-pain, toothache and arthralgia.

Hua Tuo also recommended physical exercises. He conceived a particular gymnastic exercise known as the 'movement of five animals'. It consisted of adopting the position of a tiger about to leap, of turning the head like a deer, standing erect like a bear, jumping on tiptoe like a monkey, and stretching the arms like a bird flying. Due to this exercise, according to the *Houhanshu*, Hua Tuo's disciple, Wu Pu, lived until he was ninety and was able to preserve all his faculties.

Three of Hua Tuo's disciples are well known in the history of

Chinese medicine: Wu Pu, Li Dangzhi and Fan A. Wu Pu was the author of a medical work that carried his name, *Wu Pu Bencao*.[30] Fan A is especially renowned as an acupuncturist. Finally, the authorship of the *Zhongzangjing*, a classic of traditional Chinese medicine, has been attributed to Hua Tuo, although it is extremely doubtful that he was in fact the author.[31]

An Honorarium of Apricots

Dong Feng, along with Zhang Zhongjing and Hua Tuo, has the reputation of being one of 'three extraordinary physicians of the Jian'an era', which began in AD 196 and coincided with the last years of the reign of Emperor Xian. At the end of his life, Dong Feng, like a good Daoist, retired to live in the Lu mountains, earning himself the sobriquet 'Dong the Immortal'. He adopted the unique practice of only accepting apricot-trees for payment, the number of which would vary according to the gravity of the illness. After several years, Dong Feng's collection of apricot-trees was known as 'Dong the Immortal's apricot orchard'. The expression 'apricot orchard' has been used ever since in praise of a good physician.

Notes

1. Dominique Hoizey, *Li Po: Parmi les Nuages et les Pins* (Paris: Arfuyen, 1984). The 'six directions' refers to the six states that the future Qin emperor would annex.
2. Jacques Gernet, *A History of Chinese Civilization*, op. cit., p 111. On Legalism, see Leon Vandermeersch, *La Formation du Légisme* (Paris: Ecole Française d'Extrême-Orient, 1965). Vandermeersch notes (p 274): 'The emergence of the Legalist school of thought coincided with that of Chinese caesarism, of which it was an ideological reflection'.
3. J. Lanzmann (ed.), *Dispute sur le Sel et le Fer* (Paris, 1978).
4. Anna Seidel, *La Divinisation de Lao Tseu dans la Taoisme des Han* (Paris: Ecole Française d'Extrême-Orient, 1969), p 73.
5. Danielle and Vadime Elisseeff, *La Civilisation de la Chine Classique* (Paris: Arthaud, 1979), p 186.
6. Dominique Hoizey, *Li Po: Parmi les Nuages et les Pins*, op. cit.
7. Kristofer Schipper, *L'Empereur Wou des Han dans la Légende Taoiste* (Paris: Ecole Française d'Extrême-Orient, 1965).
8. Henri Maspero, *Le Taoisme et les Religions Chinoises* (Paris: Gallimard, 1971), p 354.
9. Manfred Porkert, *Biographie d'un Taoiste Légendaire: Tcheou Tseu-yang* (Paris: Institut des Hautes Etudes Chinoises, 1979). This hagiographic text was produced after the period with which we are concerned here (it dates from the fourth century AD), although the author refers to this Daoist sage of immortality as living during the late Eastern Han dynasty.
10. Cited by Joseph Needham, *The Grand Titration*, op. cit., p 158.
11. *Zhuangzi*, op. cit., pp 196–7.
12. *Mawangdui Hanmu*, op. cit., pp 117–20.

13. *Changsha Mawangdui Yihao Hanmu* (Beijing: Wenwu Chubanshe, 1980), and, especially, *Bingli Bianhua Ji Siyin Fenxi (Analysis of Pathological Change and the Causes of Death)*, pp 267–93.
14. *Mancheng Hanmu (The Han Tombs of Mancheng)* (Beijing: Wenwu chubanshe, 1978).
15. According to the *Summary of Chinese Acupuncture* (Beijing: Foreign Language Press, 1977), p 85, when a *zang* or *fu* organ is unsettled, a morbid reaction often occurs on the *shu* point of the back. Thus gastralgia is treated by puncturing the *weishu* point (*wei*: 'stomach').
16. *Changsha Mawangdui Yihao Hanmu Chutu Dongzhiwu Biaoben De Yanjiu (Research on the Plant and Animal Specimens Exhumed from the Number One Han Tomb at Mawangdui, Changsha)* (Beijing: Wenwu Chubanshe, 1978), pp 21–42.
17. On the *Trichosanthes kirilowii*, see p 180.
18. *Shanghanlun*, translated by Catherine Despeux (Paris: Editions de la Tisserande, 1985), p 19.
19. *Wenwu*, no 12 (1973), pp 23–9.
20. Ming Wong, *Shanghanlun* (Paris: Masson, 1983), translates *shanglan* as 'noxious cold' (*shang*: 'to wound, harm'; *han*: 'cold'). Catherine Despeux prefers 'attack of cold'. The term should not be confused with *shanghan* ('typhoid fever').
21. Ming Wong, *Shanghanlun*, op. cit., p 6.
22. Catherine Despeux, op. cit., pp 33–4, gives a description of the prescription.
23. Ibid., pp 39–40.
24. Ibid., pp 43–4, 45–6.
25. Ibid., pp 131–3.
26. Ibid., p 121.
27. The debate surrounding the nationality of Hua Tuo is the subject of an article by Lang Xucai in *Zhonghua Yishi Zazhi (Chinese Journal of Medical History)*, 16:2 (April 1986).
28. The journal *Minjian Wenxue* periodically publishes anecdotes concerning Hua Tuo. See, especially, no 6 (1981), pp 43–53, and no 12 (1985), p 9. Comic strips include *Hua Tuo* (Beijing: Renmin Meishu Chubanshe, 1979), and *Zhongguo Gudai Kexuejia* (Shanghai: Renmin Chubanshe, 1977).
29. Catherine Despeux, op. cit., p 96.
30. On Wu Pu's *Materia Medica*, see Liang Maoxin's article in *Zhonghua Yishi Zazhi (Chinese Journal of Medical History)*, no 3 (1986), pp 177–82, and *Wu Pu Bencao* (Beijing: Renmin Weisheng Chubanshe, 1987).
31. *Zhongzangjing*, revised and annotated by Wu Changguo (Nanjing: Jiangsu Kexue Jishu Chubanshe, 1985).

4

From the Three Kingdoms to the Northern and Southern Dynasties, 220–589

The Chinese 'Middle Ages'[1]

The 400-year period from the fall of the Han dynasty to the succession of the Sui dynasty is so complex that it would be foolhardy to give a detailed summary. China was initially under the military control of the Three Kingdoms (Wei, Shu-Han, Wu), which divided the empire between AD 220 and 280. Dominant personalities acquired fame during these years, such as Cao Cao (d. 220), the founder of the Wei kingdom in north China, and Zhuge Liang (d. 234), adviser to Liu Bei, a descendant of the Han emperors who founded the kingdom of Shu-Han in Sichuan. The Western Jin dynasty (265–317), which took over from the kingdom of Wu in 280 and was established at Luoyang and then Nanjing, was succeeded by the eastern Jin (317–420), one of the five dynasties (Eastern Jin, Song, Qi, Liang and Chen) that ruled over southern China (the Yangzi basin) until 589. North China came under the sway of the Northern Wei dynasty (386–584), established by the Tabgatch (or Tuoba), which embraced the Chinese culture and way of life.

Jacques Gernet underlines the profound differences separating northern Chinese society of the fourth century – 'warlike, non-elitist, almost illiterate, and influenced by the cultures of the steppe and the Sino-Tibetan frontier region' – from southern Chinese society centred on the Yangzi basin, which was 'aristocratic and sophisticated'. Yet he also notes that 'Buddhism was propagated with equal enthusiasm throughout the early Chinese world'.[2] The China of this period was, above all else, Buddhist. Moreover, the Northern Wei dynasty depended on this new religion to consolidate its power. This was a time when 'natural' sanctuaries were created, such as the Buddhist caves of Yungang near Datong, the Northern Wei capital until 494. This sculpted cliff-side, one of the most beautiful 'cathedrals' of Buddhist China, embodied the unity of the

49

empire deriving from the person of the emperor, the 'living Buddha'. A parallel can be made with the France of Suger, where the abbey of Saint-Denis was seen as symbolising the authority of the king, 'vicar of God'. In south China, on the other hand, the monk Huiyuan (334–416), one of the most significant personalities of the fourth and fifth centuries, was the advocate for Buddhism's independence vis-à-vis the secular power.

The propagation of Buddhism, expeditions to India by Chinese monks (such as Faxian in the early fifth century) and the arrival in China of Indian monks (such as Paramartha, a prolific translator of the sixth century) all contributed to the spread of Indian culture throughout the Chinese world. It influenced such diverse branches of learning as mathematics, astronomy and medicine. This influence is clearly evident in the case of Tao Hongjing, a late convert to Buddhism; one of his medical works evoked the Buddhist concept of the '101 ailments'. Other foreign contributions (from Japan and Korea) to Chinese medicine and pharmacy, in exchange for which China offered its own knowledge, cannot be overlooked. Commercial relations with far-off Arab countries facilitated the introduction there of Chinese alchemy at the height of its development. Its most renowned representative is Ge Hong, of whom more will be said later because of his major contribution to the development of Chinese medicine and pharmacy.

Daoism, medicine and alchemy are so closely linked in China that it would be difficult to doubt, as Joseph Needham notes, 'that Arab experimenters and writers were profoundly influenced by Chinese concepts and discoveries, hardly less so perhaps than they were by Greek techniques of producing gold preserved by Byzantine culture'.[3] It has been observed, in fact, that alchemy in Arab culture, as in Chinese culture, was marked by medical concerns. Whatever the case, from the end of the Han to the Northern and Southern Dynasties, Daoist adepts persevered with their quest for longevity and with research into the processes, alchemical or otherwise, that would accomplish such a result. The key stage involved in alchemy was the consumption of cinnabar (*dan*, from which is derived the expression *liandanshu*, meaning 'art or technique of purifying cinnabar'), but considerable preparation was required beforehand. Ge Hong, the noted alchemist of this period, speaks in the *Baopuzi* of transmuting (*zhuan*) cinnabar nine times to achieve sublimation.

Alchemy promoted the development of pharmaceutical science which, judging by the number of works listed in the *Suishu* (*History of the Sui*), took on a new lease of life during this period. In particular, one such work listed was the edition of *Shen'nong*

Bencaojing revised by Tao Hongjing at the beginning of the sixth century. The experiments carried out by alchemists, in particular those of Ge Hong, during the fourth century paved the way for the emergence of a chemical pharmacy. During the fifth century, in fact, a work appeared specifically devoted to the manufacture of medicines, the first of its kind in the history of Chinese pharmacy.

As a result of war and the need to treat its victims, surgical practice greatly improved, and it is no coincidence that the first Chinese text on surgery was written at this time. Another significant feature of the Chinese 'Middle Ages' was the establishment of formal medical instruction. Hitherto, medical knowledge had been passed on from master to pupil, but in 443 Qin Chengzu, a physician serving the emperor of the Song (one of the Southern Dynasties), proposed the creation of a school of medicine.

Wang Shuhe, the Promoter of Pulsing

The familiar image of the patient, facing a physician across a small table and holding out his wrist, illustrates the importance that Chinese traditional medicine has always attached to examination of the pulse. It is considered essential in arriving at a diagnosis; rather than calculating the number of pulse-beats per minute, however, it is more a way of disclosing, as Jacques-André Lavier emphasises, the qualitative aspect of any palpitation:

> Western physiologists have for a long time noticed that the beating of the pulse does not result from the circulatory process itself, but from the extremely rapid transmission of impulses along the vascular walls. It is precisely these impulses that bear the features of what is here in question.[4]

Namely these are symptoms of an illness that cannot always be clinically anticipated and that ultimately have to be deliberately induced. Thus, according to the *Shanghanlun*, if 'the patient has a floating and moderate pulse, does not feel any bodily aches, but his body feels heavy and light in turn . . . one has to induce the symptoms of the illness'.[5] The nature of the pulse can determine the action to be taken. Thus Zhang Zhongjing strongly advises that 'when a patient with symptoms of a chest congestion has a floating and high pulse, do not carry out purging since this will cause death'.[6] When Hua Tuo attended to General Li's wife, it was by taking her pulse that he was able to confirm his diagnosis with assurance: 'Her pulse is the same; there are indeed two foetuses; the first has lost much blood, preventing the second from being expelled'.

Drawing on the experience of his predecessors, Wang Shuhe

(who lived in the third century) compiled the *Maijing* (*Pulse Classic*), which brought together all the knowledge accumulated in this area since the compilation of the *Huangdi Neijing*. The *Maijing* is thus the earliest Chinese treatise on pulsing. It differentiated twenty-four kinds of pulse, among which were floating (*fu*), smooth (*hua*), tense (*jin*), deep (*chen*), unstable (*ge*), faint (*wei*), uneven (*se*), fine (*xi*), tremulous (*dong*), weak (*ruo*) and moderate (*huan*). A floating and shallow pulse is visible to the eye, explains Jacques-André Lavier, so that it is like a natural river; on the other hand, a deep and hard pulse 'gives the impression of feeling a small stone at the bottom of a shallow river'.[7] The *Maijing* also refers to the three radial positions for examining the pulse: the anterior pulse (*cun*: 'inch'), which is nearest the hand, the middle pulse (*guan*: 'bar'), which is situated between the other two, and the posterior pulse (*chi*: 'cubit'), the furthest from the hand. In addition to compiling the *Maijing*, Wang Shuhe was also responsible for reconstructing the text of the *Shanghanlun*, of which only a few fragments had survived.

Huangfu Mi and his *ABC of Acupuncture*

Acupuncture is regarded as a national treasure in China, and Huangfu Mi (215–82), the celebrated author of *Zhenjiu Jiayijing* (*The ABC of Acupuncture and Moxibustion*), inherited a valuable tradition bequeathed by his predecessors. The *Lingshu*, a section of the *Huangdi Neijing*, also known as the *Zhenjing* (*Book of Acupuncture*), was further enriched by several centuries of practice. Qin Yueren, Zhang Zhongjing and Hua Tuo often resorted to acupuncture and moxibustion as part of their therapy. The *Houhanshu* (*History of the Later Han*) relates that Hua Tuo cured Cao Cao's migraine through the use of acupuncture, while the same source notes that Fan A, one of Hua Tuo's disciples, succeeded in puncturing the back by one or two inches and the thorax by five to six inches.[8] Moreover, a series of acupuncture points covering the two sides of the vertebral column are named after Hua Tuo.[9]

Huangfu Mi's humble origins did not suggest the prospect of a brilliant official career, medical or otherwise, but a niggling rheumatism from which he began to suffer at the age of forty induced him to study medicine. Thereafter he devoted the rest of his life to this vocation, although he continued to maintain an interest in literature and history. Although known as a poet, writer and historian, Huangfu Mi's name is principally associated with the *Zhenjiu Jiayijing*, which has exerted considerable influence on succeeding generations of practitioners both in China and abroad, especially Japan.

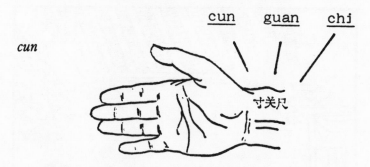

cun

FIGURE 4.1   From *Zhongyixue Jichu* (Beijing: Renmin Weisheng Chubanshe, 1984).

Huangfu Mi's greatest merit was to have gathered together in one text all previous knowledge and experience in the domain of acupuncture acquired since the *Huangdi Neijing*. He relied on the *Suwen*, the *Zhenjing* and the *Mingdang Kongxue Zhenjiu Zhiyao*, aiming to 'cut out inconsistent observations and repetitions'. He also took into account his own observations in compiling the *ABC of Acupuncture*, which, in effect, is the earliest summary of acupuncture and moxibustion.

The work begins with references to traditional concepts of Chinese medicine in the fields of anatomy and physiology, before outlining the theory and nature of the meridians (the twelve regular channels and the eight 'extraordinary' channels) and then describing the various acupuncture points and their therapeutic qualities. The technique of manipulating the needles (the extent of penetration for example) is dealt with, as is the clinical application of acupuncture and moxibustion.

Ge Hong, Alchemist and Physician

Ge Hong (c. 281–341) has been described as 'the leading light of his generation in the realm of science literature'.[10] This multitalented scholar, in fact, contributed much to the development of Chinese science during the first half of the fourth century. As an alchemist and Daoist adept in search of drugs to prolong life, his experiments opened the way for the development of chemical pharmacy, while his notions of medicine as recorded in the *Zhouhou Beijifang* (*Emergency Prescriptions*) demonstrate a pragmatic approach to therapy, with particular attention paid to preventive measures.

Known also by the pseudonym of Baopuzi, Ge Hong was a native of Jurong district in Jiangsu province. His father died when he was

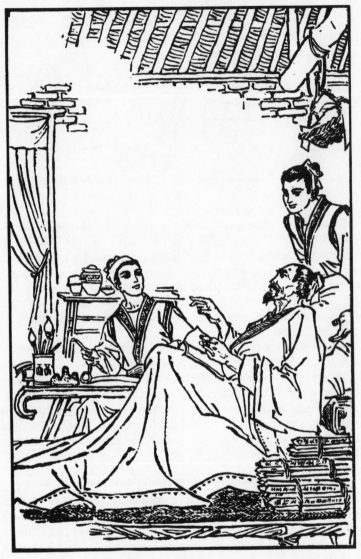

FIGURE 4.2   Huangfu Mi. From *Zhongguo Gudai Yixuejia De Gushi*
(Shanghai: Shaonian Ertong Chubanshe, 1979).

thirteen, and several years later he embarked on a study of the Confucian classics and various other works. It may have been his Confucian education that prompted Ge Hong to support the Western Jin dynasty in its suppression of a peasant insurrection. The writer Lu Xun once observed that 'those who put Confucius on a pedestal are the people in power or those who thirst for power. Confucius is their sage, a sage who has no relevance for the masses.'[11] Whatever the case, after several reversals of fortune due to the insecurity of the times, Ge Hong finally settled in Guangzhou (Canton), his talents as yet having brought little success.

The grand-nephew of Ge Xuan, a Daoist of the Three Kingdoms period, Ge Hong was twenty when he was introduced to alchemy by a disciple of his great-uncle, Zheng Yin. When he arrived in Guangzhou, Ge Hong had already mastered alchemical techniques. In Guangzhou, he pursued his research with Bao Xuan as his teacher. The ascension to power in 317 of Sima Rui, founder of the Eastern Jin dynasty, gave him the opportunity of returning to his native district. Eventually, however, he gave up his official post awarded for past services and retired to Mount Luofu in Guangdong.

Inspired by the desire to prolong human life, and therefore preoccupied with 'nourishing the vital principle' (yangsheng), Ge Hong turned to alchemy. It has been emphasised earlier, quoting Joseph Needham, that one of the factors assisting the development of Chinese alchemy was 'the absence of any prejudice against the use of mineral drugs'. In his experiments, details of which are recorded in one of his written works, the Bupaozi, Ge Hong not only worked with cinnabar, the principal substance for Chinese alchemists, but also with many other minerals such as realgar, sulphur, steatite, saltpetre, alum, lodestone, mica, iron and tin. Although Ge Hong was versed in the processes of sublimation and distillation, it is the therapeutic aspect of his experiments that especially attracts our attention. In addition to mineral drugs, the Bupaozi refers to medicinal plants that are still used today: the resin of the conifer, the rhizome of the Rehmannia glutinosa, the root of the Liriope spicata, rhizomes of the Coptis chinensis and Polygonatum sibiricum, and a certain kind of mushroom, Poria cocos.[12]

The Zhouhou Beijifang (Emergency Prescriptions) is like a medical handbook that aims to be both practical and effective. Ge Hong intended to give all the means possible for the quickest and cheapest cure, proposing the use of readily accessible and inexpensive drugs. He also recommended therapeutic measures such as acupuncture and moxibustion. Other recommendations included the 'horn method' (treatment by cupping),[13] massage, and cure by fumigation. A number of drugs prescribed by Ge Hong are still used today to treat the same illnesses: *Dichroa febrifuga* to combat malaria, *Ephedra sinica* to combat asthma, and the arsenic of natural sulphur (realgar) to combat various skin ailments.

The *Zhouhou Beijifang* lists the diseases of the time: typhoid, dysentery, malaria, erysipelas, smallpox, leprosy and cholera. The symptoms of each are described, sometimes rather arbitrarily, such as in the case of leprosy, where the patient 'initially feels that his skin is numb, or feels itchy as if insects were darting under his skin, or else sees things through his skin as if it were suspended silk', and sometimes with more precision such as in the case of smallpox or of an ailment peculiar to East Asia known as 'Japanese river fever' (which Ge Hong designates as 'sand-lice disease'), a form of rickets caused by the *Rickettsia tsutsugamushi* or *Rickettsia orientalis*. Ge Hong was clearly unaware of the existence of this micro-organism (referred to as rickets), but he observed in detail the causes and symptoms of this disease caused by the bite of the 'sand flea' (*shashi*). We know today that the fever is transmitted to humans through two species of red mullet (*Trombicula delhiensis* and *Trombicula akamushi*). Ge Hong gives a clinical description of the symptoms that is identical to that given today – fever, body-aches and skin rash.

Preventive measures were another of Ge Hong's concerns, and he recommended the use of prophylactic drugs and the quarantine of patients with contagious diseases.

Tao Hongjing, Commentator of the *Shen'nong Bencaojing*

Like Ge Hong a native of Jiangsu, Tao Hongjing (456–536) lived during the first three Southern Dynasties (Song, Qi, Liang), which followed one another between 420 and 557. Tao had numerous interests which led him to study medicine, astronomy and geography, although he excelled equally in other fields as diverse as music, chess and calligraphy. After his conversion to Buddhism, Tao led the life of a recluse.

Tao Hongjing is especially renowned as the commentator of the *Shen'nong Bencaojing*, which he revised and annotated, increasing the number of herbal drugs listed to 730 and giving more detailed information on their nature, location and the particular time when the plants should be gathered. Tao's *Shen'nong Bencaojing Jizhu* (*Annotations to the Classic of Herbal Medicine*) dominated Chinese pharmaceutical literature until the middle of the seventh century.

It is to Tao Hongjing that we also owe the completion of Ge Hong's *Zhouhou Beijifang*, which became the *Zhouhou Baiyi Fang* (*101 Emergency Prescriptions*). How was a work such as this transmitted? The prescriptions recommended by Ge Hong, Tao Hongjing and other, anonymous, therapists were often copied by hand and then circulated, although sometimes they were engraved on stone in places such as the famous Buddhist caves of Longmen (Dragon's Gate), to the south of Loyang in Henan province. The 100 or so 'prescriptions of Dragon's Gate' were engraved in one of the caves of this noted Buddhist site towards the end of the sixth century. The proposed cures are for infectious diseases such as malaria (to be treated, as recommended also by Ge Hong, with *Dichroa febrifuga*), as well as for less serious ailments such as simple indigestion.

Chinese pharmacy owes much to Tao Hongjing for providing it with an innovative impulse that was to bear fruit during the Tang dynasty. Two other figures of the period deserve to share this recognition. Xu Zhicai (505–72) classified drugs in terms of their effectiveness, while Lei Xiao (born in the fifth century) wrote the earliest Chinese work on galenic pharmacy (preparation of vegetable-based medicine as opposed to chemical remedies), the *Lei Gong Baozhilun* (*Treatise on the Preparation of Lei Gong's Remedies*). It describes various ways of preparing medicine, such as steaming (*zheng*), boiling (*zhu*) or heating over an open fire (*bao*).

The Surgeon Gong Qingxuan

Fu Weikang observes that 'surgery in China, as with medicine, has a long history'.[14] The first Chinese 'surgeons' who used the celebrated stone slivers (*bian*) in order to make skin incisions (the *Huangdi Neijing* notes that such incisions aimed to cure abscesses) were succeeded by a number of legendary figures whose skills were sometimes exaggerated. Qin Yueren, for example, was said to have carried out heart transplants. On the other hand, it is perfectly credible that Chunyi Yi treated injuries to the lower back. Also, we know from the *Houhanshu* (*History of the Later Han*) that Hua Tuo carried out laparotomy during the latter half of the second century.

The *Jinshu* (*History of the Jin Dynasty*) notes that a physician of the fifth century operated on a man afflicted with hare-lip. About the same period, Gong Qingxuan (end of the fifth century?) recorded the procedures carried out by a certain Liu Juanzi, who had lived during the fifth century. This work, known by the title of *Liu Juanzi Guiyifang*, is the oldest Chinese treatise on surgery. It provides a wealth of information on the experiences gained up to the fifth century in the treatment of wounds caused by metal instruments (in particular steel weapons) and of ailments affecting the skin such as boils, anthrax and abscesses. The use of mercurial ointment is mentioned in the cure of skin illnesses.[15]

Notes

1. The term is borrowed from Jacques Gernet, *A History of Chinese Civilization*, op. cit., p 172.
2. Ibid., pp 174–85.
3. Joseph Needham, *The Grand Titration*, op. cit., p 69.
4. Jacques-André Lavier, *Médecine Chinoise, Médecine Totale* (Paris: Grasset, 1973), p 126.
5. Catherine Despeux, op. cit., p 47.
6. Ibid., p 77.
7. Jacques-André Lavier, op. cit., p 132.
8. The *cun* ('inch') is a measure of length used in acupuncture. One can understand the prudence shown by predecessors of Hua Tuo and Fan A, since the *Summary of Chinese Acupuncture* (op. cit., p 18) recommends that 'as the skin tissue of certain areas of the thorax is soft, if not thin, and as the acupuncture points located in these areas are close to important organs such as the heart, lungs, liver and spleen, it is advisable not to puncture the skin too deeply and for the needle to be inserted in a slanting, almost horizontal, direction'.
9. A description of this procedure can be found in the *Summary of Chinese Acupuncture*, op. cit., pp 213–14.
10. Manfred Porkert, *Biographie d'un Taoist Légendaire*, op. cit., p 3.
11. Lu Xun 'Confucius dans la Chine moderne', in *Lu Xun: Pamphlets et Libelles (1925–1936)*, introduced and translated by Michelle Loi (Paris: François Maspero, 1977), pp 208–15.
12. The rhizome of the *Coptis chinensis* (belonging to the family of ranunculus), used to combat fever and dysentery, contains berberine, which is much used in China today for its antimicrobial properties. See Xiao Peigen's report at the international congress on therapeutic plants and natural substances, held in Monastir (Tunisia), 7–9 May 1986.
13. This treatment is recommended today to cure a number of afflictions: lesions of the joints, aches in the limbs, and asthma. See *Summary of Chinese Acupuncture*, op. cit., pp 33–4.
14. Fu Weikang, 'Surgery in Ancient Chinese Medicine', in *Traditional Chinese Medicine and Pharmacology* (Beijing: Foreign Language Press, 1985), p 75.
15. Jean-Claude Dousset, *Histoire des Médicaments* (Paris: Payot, 1985), p 118, notes that the well-known physician of the Renaissance, Ambroise Paré, recommended the use of mercurial ointment in the treatment of syphilis.

— 5 —

The Sui and Tang Empires, 581–907

A Restored Unity

'Sooner or later, the idea re-emerged that the dispersal of power in China had to give way once more to the national unity characteristic of earlier, more glorious, periods of the country's history',[1] write D. and V. Elisseeff in their introduction to the 'second classical period' (the first being that of the Han) of the Sui and Tang dynasties. The accession to power of the Sui dynasty in 581, followed in 589 by the overthrow of the last of the Southern Dynasties (Chen), represented the culmination of the 'northern' dream of national unity that had led a general of the Northern Zhou dynasty (557–81) to take power and establish a new dynasty, adopting the reign title of Sui Wendi. According to historians, the megalomania of his successor, Sui Yangdi, led to the overthrow of the infant dynasty. What is certain is that the dynasty was confronted with serious problems such as peasant revolts and the burden of military campaigns against Korea. It was at this time that the Li family entered the political scene. The patriarch, Li Yuan, and his son, Li Shimin, rebelled against the Sui and founded the Tang dynasty. They reigned under the names of Tang Gaozu (618–26) and Tang Taizong (626–49) respectively.

The first Tang emperors completed the work of the Sui, which had built cities (Chang'an and Luoyang) and waterways, and undertook a programme of reorganisation in the administrative, judicial, economic and military spheres. They also undertook a large offensive in 630 against the threatening Turks; this was the beginning of a huge expansion which was to make early Tang China of the seventh century the most powerful country in Asia. The end of the seventh and beginning of the eighth centuries were marked by the dominant personality of Empress Wu who, on Tang Gaozong's death in 683, assumed the title of 'emperor' and reigned under the name of Zetian ('conforming with heaven'). Historical judgment on her role has been very mixed, and one Chinese historian does not hesitate in describing her as one of China's 'female calamities'. Her rival was the Empress Wei, wife of Emperor Zhongzong, whom she had poisoned in 710.

The eighth century was dominated by the figure of Emperor Xuanzong (712–56). The Kaiyuan period (713–41), especially, was one of prosperity, evoked with nostalgia by the poet Du Fu (712–70), who referred to the joyous time when 'neither jackals nor tigers were to be seen on the roads throughout the nine regions'.

The rebellion of An Lushan in 755 brought this 'golden age' to an abrupt end. China was thrown into a state of warfare described by another great poet of the period, Li Bai (701–62), in verses tinged with sadness:

> Casting my eyes on the plain of Luoyang
> I see a Tartar army through the mist
> The wild grass is red with spilt blood
> And wolves and jackals don official caps.[2]

In the following century, Bai Juyi (772–846) wrote a poem on the love between Emperor Xuanzong and the beautiful concubine Yang Guifei, who, in 756, was given up to the generals clamouring for her death:

> Of the 3,000 beauties in the palace
> She alone was lavished with the 3,000 favours.[3]

After 755, the Tang entered a period of decline. Imperial appointees who commanded military garrisons took advantage of their increased powers as a result of the frequent rebellions that broke out at the end of the ninth century. Their enhanced power, in conjunction with eunuch intrigues at court, led to division and disorder.

The Tang era has been described as China's 'second classical period'. Chinese civilisation at this time attained one of its high peaks. In particular, it was a time when there was an extraordinary outburst of poetic talent and when Buddhist influence in China reached its zenith. The *Quantangshi* (*Complete Collection of Tang Poems*), published in 1705, comprises 48,900 poems by 2,300 poets. Li Bai, Du Fu and Bai Juyi have already been mentioned; other celebrated names include Meng Haoran (689–740), Wang Wei (701–61), Du Mu (803–52) and Li Shangyin (813–58). Buddhism, as a foreign religion, underwent a long process of sinicisation and was profoundly influenced by Confucianism and Daoism. The most specifically Chinese school of Buddhiam, *Chan* (or *Zen* in Japanese), which appeared in China towards the end of the fifth century, particularly thrived during the Tang dynasty. The school boasted exceptional masters such as Huineng (638–713), Mazu Daoyi (709–88), Huangbo (ninth century) and Linji (ninth century). Moreover, it survived the anti-Buddhist persecutions of the mid-ninth century. Translations of Indian Buddhist texts increased in number, notably through the initiative of Xuanzang (seventh century), a monk whose pilgrimage to India has become famous.

The Medical Centre of Asia

Medicine and pharmacy, enriched by new experiences, witnessed a rapid growth during the Tang. A reading of medical and pharmaceutical works during this period reveals the level of development attained in these two fields during the course of the three centuries considered one of the most brilliant periods in Chinese history. Aetiology and semiology were important beneficiaries of this progress, as can be seen in the *Zhubingyuan Houlun* (*Treatise on the Causes and Symptoms of Illness*) compiled by Chao Yuanfang at the beginning of the seventh century. The work discusses the risk of infection from wounds as well as the causes for parasitic diseases such as tapeworm, which, according to Chao Yuanfang, originated with the consumption of uncooked beef.[4] For his part, Sun Simiao recommended that his contemporaries seek an alimentary cause for cholera rather than blame a malevolent spirit, an attitude that Bai Juyi in the ninth century condemns in ironic verse:

> Whenever famine, flood, drought or illness occurs
> That is the time villagers blame the dragon.[5]

At the same time, various preventive measures were adopted. Hospitals for lepers made their appearance, and ways were sought to guard against rabies, smallpox and typhoid. On the pharmaceutical front, the Tang dynasty was a rich period for *bencao*, treatises on herbal medicine of which the most celebrated is the *Xinxiu Bencao* (*Newly-revised Herbal Medicine*), also known as the *Tang Bencao* (*Herbal Medicine of the Tang*), the first official Chinese pharmacopoeia. Manuals on the cultivation and harvesting of medicinal plants were also produced, as well as various other specialist works such as the *Hu Bencao* (*Tartar Herbal Medicine*), an example of the contribution made by non-Chinese peoples to the development of medicine and pharmacy, particularly in the domain of phytotherapy.

The very name of Tang itself brings to mind a China open to

foreign influences but which also 'exported' its own knowledge and skills. Only the exchanges concerned with medicine and pharmacy will be dealt with here, although China's relations with Japan, Korea, Vietnam, India and Persia brought in their wake many other cultural developments, as the following account of the Buddhist monk, Jianzhen, shows.

Jianzhen was born in 688 at Yangzhou with the family name of Chunyu. He entered the monastic life from adolescence and several years later travelled to Chang'an and Luoyang to study Buddhist doctrines, architecture, fine arts and medicine. On returning to Yangzhou, he took charge of the Daming temple. His reputation became known by two Japanese Buddhist missionaries in Chang'an, who invited him to Japan. After several attempts, Jianzhen finally reached Japan in 753. He died in Nara in 763.

Jianzhen had a considerable influence in Japan, not only in the realm of Buddhist doctrine itself but also in the fields of architecture, fine arts, literature, calligraphy, wood-engraving and medicine. He was particularly versed in the study of herbal medicine, so much so that after he became blind he was able to recognise a medicinal plant by its odour, touch and taste. In his youth, Jianzhen had received a Buddhist education that was drawn from the *pancavidya*, the 'five sciences' in India of which medicine (*cikitsa*) was a component. Moreover, the town of Yangzhou was renowned for its medical instruction. Jianzhen practised medicine there in between preaching, devoting some of his time to the cure of patients who frequented the temple dispensary. His medical knowledge, particularly in the realm of phytotherapy, enhanced his reputation in Japan, where he was long accorded much respect.

Sino-Korean relations flourished during the Tang, allowing the introduction into Korea of the classics of Chinese medicine and even more contemporary works such as Chao Yuanfang's *Zhubing Yuanhoulun* or Sun Simiao's *Qianjin Yaofang* (*Prescriptions of the Thousand Ounces of Gold*). At the same time, Korean herbal medicine was introduced to China.

Herbal medicine (*bencao*) was also enriched with plant species of Vietnamese origin such as *Aquilaria agollocha*, a tree with a fragrant wood whose 'leaves and bark are utilised in the making of perfumed paper',[6] *Liquidamber orientalis* and various other aromatic plants.

Through the influence of Buddhism, it became fashionable to seek knowledge of India. Numerous expeditions there were undertaken via 'the western countries'. The most famous of such journeys was that of Xuanzang in the seventh century. The account

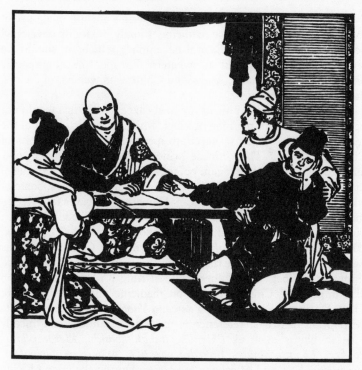

FIGURE 5.1   Jianzhen giving medical advice. From *Jianzhen Heshang* (Shanghai: Renmin Meishu Chubanshe, 1979).

of this journey, *Datang Xiyuji* (*A Record of the Western Countries during the Tang*), provides a wealth of information on India at this time. Indian medical works were translated into Chinese, and Indian physicians even practised in China. Chinese ophthalmology benefited from the Indian experience while, in turn, India received from China medicinal plants such as ginseng, angelica and the ephedra.

Arab medicine was able to borrow from China not only alchemy (the origin of medical chemistry) but also pulsology; Wang Shuhe's *Maijing* (*The Pulse Classic*) appears to have had a particular influence in this domain. There is evidence of Chinese contributions to Arab medicine in the *Book of Medicine* by Avicenna (980–1037). Due to expanding commercial relations during the Tang, Arab merchants were able to introduce China to incense, myrrh and fenugreek (*Trigonella foenum-graecum*), while from Persia came the fig (*Ficus carica*) whose laxative properties are still made use of today in traditional Chinese medicine. Finally, relations developed between China and the Byzantine empire, which, it should be remembered, transmitted to western Europe 'the therapeutic practices of the Persians, Arabs and Chinese as well as, of course, the Greeks and Romans'.[7]

This description of China as the medical centre of Asia would not be complete without mention of Tibet, which in the latter half of the seventh century 'began to succumb increasingly to the charms of Chinese culture'.[8] The Chinese princess Wencheng, who in 641 married King Sron btsan sgam po, took with her not only a statue of the Buddha Sakyamuni but also various medical writings, some of which were translated into Tibetan. Chinese physicians followed in the steps of Princess Wencheng and travelled to Tibet. One such physician was Han Wenhai; during his sojourn, he wrote the *Handi Zabing Zhiliao* (*The Art of Curing Patients the Chinese Way*) as well as helping to compile the *Wuwei Wuqi*, which was distributed throughout Tibet. The Chinese wife of King K'ri lde gtsug brtsan also introduced Chinese works on medicine and pharmacy into Tibet. During this period, the *Yuewang Yaozhen* was written; in its description of drugs, reference is made to a number of typically Tibetan plants such as *Phlomis younghusbandii, Pterocephalus hookeri, Lagotis glauca, Ephedra saxatilis, Aconitum naviculare, Veronica ciliata* and *Mirabalis himalaica*. During the reign of King K'ri sron lde brtsan in the latter half of the eighth century, Tibetan medicine, benefiting from the cooperation with Chinese and Indian physicians, underwent further development and was enriched with newly-translated medical works.

At the same time, among the Uighur people in Xinjiang, medicine became more advanced; it would later be influenced by the theories of Avicenna.

Medical instruction itself during the Tang was the responsibility of the Imperial Bureau of Medicine (*Taiyishu*), the central agency for the administration and teaching of medicine. It had two departments, one for medicine and the other for pharmacy. The former was divided into four sections: medicine, acupuncture, massage and 'incantations'. This last 'speciality' arose from the influence of Daoism and Buddhism, but its psychological function should not be overlooked. Medical instruction dealt with internal medicine, surgery and paediatrics, as well as otorhinolaryngology and ophthalmology, and relied on such works as the *ABC of Acupuncture and Moxibustion* by Huangmi Fu and the *Maijing* (*Pulse Classic*) by Wang Shuhe. The department of pharmacy maintained a botanical garden where students could familiarise themselves with medicinal plants.

Chao Yuanfang, Aetiologist and Semiologist

Chao Yuanfang, active between the sixth and seventh centuries, can be considered the most significant medical figure during the Sui dynasty. He wrote an important work on aetiology and semiology, the *Zhubing Yuanhoulun* (*Treatise on the Causes and Symptoms of Maladies*). Drawing on the tradition represented by the *Huangdi Neijing*, the *Nanjing*, the *Shanghanlun* and the *Jingui Yaolue*, the book exerted a profound influence on the future development of Chinese medicine. Chao himself occupied the post of *taiyi* (physician to the emperor).

The illnesses examined in the *Zhubing Yuanhoulun* depend principally for their treatment on internal medicine, surgery, gynaecology, paediatrics, otorhinolaryngology, ophthalmology and dermatology. The book also gives details on infectious and contagious diseases such as smallpox, measles, scarlet fever, tuberculosis, leprosy and parasitic afflictions such as the various forms of helminthiasis (a condition characterised by the presence of worms in the body), ascariasis (threadworm), taeniasis (tapeworm) and oxyuriasis. Chao compared the blotchy exanthema (rash) associated with scarlet fever to a brocade; pointed out that smallpox pustules would leave scars; and gave a detailed description of the skin lesions caused by leprosy, in particular the mutilations caused by leprous tubercles: 'The eyelashes and eyebrows drop out . . . and the bones of the nose weaken . . .'. In the case of cerebral haemorrhage, he emphasised the trauma of an apoplectic stroke, loss of speech, and the body's rigidity. The formation of calculi (stony concretions) in the body was not overlooked. Chao spoke of 'liquid (*shui*: "water") being transformed into stone (*shi*)', what is known today as renal lithiasis (formation of stony concretions in the bladder and urinary passages). Chao equally understood the pathogenic role of the sarcoptid (itch-mite), whose presence he observed in the 'small abscesses', grooves that the itch-mite burrowed in the skin. According to Chao, this 'worm' (*chong*) could be 'extracted with the point of a needle'.[9] In the field of ophthalmology, the *Zhubing Yuanhoulun* pointed to various problems leading to diminution or loss of vision such as xerophthalmia, an inflammation of the conjunctiva with abnormal dryness ('withered eye' in Chinese). The work also refers to rickets. Finally, Chao Yuanfang mentions teeth extractions, abortions and anastomosis (cross-communication between arteries and veins).

Sun Simiao, the 'King of Prescriptions'

Sun Simiao (581–682), a native of Shanxi province, is one of the most popular figures in the history of Chinese medicine. After introducing himself to the 'three doctrines' (Confucianism, Daoism and Buddhism), in which he delighted throughout his life, the self-taught Sun turned his attention to medicine. The origins of this decision no doubt lie with his fragile health, which brought considerable expense to his parents. Sun resolved to study and practise medicine out of both necessity and a genuine attraction. In addressing his own health, he became his first patient. Sun's biography also reveals his attitude towards rulers; he turned down the tempting offers of employment proposed by Emperor Wen of the Sui and Emperors Taizong and Gaozong of the Tang, preferring the life of a humble rural physician to one that brought wealth and prestige.

The portrait of the ideal physician that Sun imagined in his writings reflected the 'humanist' notions shaped by his contact with the Confucian classics, Daoist philosophy and Buddhist teachings. According to Sun, every good physician should study the Confucian Five Classics (which included the *Book of Changes* and the *Classic of Odes* referred to earlier). If not, 'he will not know the way of *ren* and *yi*', that is the virtues of benevolence and righteousness advocated by Confucius. Neither should the ideal physician overlook the ancient philosophers and the thought of Laozi and Zhuangzi; awareness of divination and astrology was also required. In carrying out his vocation, the physician should be compassionate, and whether his patient was 'of high or low rank, wealthy or poor, adult or child, educated or illiterate, engaging or repellent, Chinese or foreigner, intelligent or foolish, the patient should be treated with the same consideration as a near relative'. Moreover, the ideal physician laboured day and night, ignoring the cold, heat, hunger, thirst and fatigue. It was with 'all his heart' that he tended to the patient. The views which Sun Simiao held of the physician's role and of medicine were not dissimilar to those inherent in Buddhism, which was very influential at this time. One need only think of the attention which Buddhism paid to the pain of existence. On the theoretical level as well, Sun Simiao drew on the Indian notion of the 'four important elements' (earth, water, fire and wind) that constituted body-matter and whose lack of equilibrium caused the 101 illnesses.

Sun Simiao's thought and practice are known through two works he wrote: *Qianjin Yaofang* (*Prescriptions of the Thousand Ounces of Gold*) and *Qianjin Yifang* (*Supplement*). The word 'gold' (*jin*) reflects the spirit in which Sun Simiao practised medicine. He considered, in fact, that all human life was a precious commodity. This champion of man's humanity contributed enormously to the development of Chinese medicine. As the inheritor of a venerable tradition, Sun was able to draw upon the medical knowledge accumulated over centuries and to enrich it with his own observations. In the *Qianjin Yaofang*, one finds reference to celebrated remedies such as decoctions of *Cinnamomum cassia* and *Ephedra sinica* prescribed by Sun's illustrious predecessor Zhang Zhongjing. Sun Simiao also had a predilection for the *Shanghanlun*, from which he borrowed copiously. Like Catherine Despeux, one might add, in fact, that Sun Simiao bequeathed a version of the *Shanghanlun* that is 'less altered than those versions we have at hand today'.[10]

With regard to herbal medicine, Sun insisted in the *Qianjin Yifang* on the need to harvest medicinal plants in the proper season and on the appropriate ways of conserving such plants and transforming them into medicine. The work lists more than 700 drugs classified according to origin: mineral (*yushi*: literally 'jade and stone'), plant (*cao*: 'herbs'), animal, insect, fish, fruit, vegetable and cereal. Sun maintained the distinction outlined in the *Shen'nong Bencaojing* among superior, average and inferior drugs for minerals and 'herbs' (i.e. plants other than fruits, vegetables and cereals). His knowledge of medical substances, particularly those of medicinal plants, earned him the nickname 'the king of medicinal herbs' or 'the king of prescriptions'.

Sun accorded therapeutic value equally to acupuncture and moxibustion, going so far as to declare: 'Acupuncture without moxibustion or vice versa is not suitable treatment. Acupuncture and moxibustion without the use of drugs or vice versa is not suitable treatment either.' What *was* suitable treatment in Sun's view was the harmonious combination of acupuncture and drugs. His diagnostic procedure relied on the four traditional examinations (observation, listening, interrogating the patient and taking the pulse) first laid down by Qin Yueren. However, Sun considered that taking the pulse had to take place after listening to the patient, beginning with his voice (*ting*: 'listen'; *sheng*: 'sound, voice'), and observing the facial complexion (*cha*: 'examine'; *se*: 'complexion'). He also attributed much importance to anticipatory diagnosis, the ideal being to cure an illness before it actually revealed itself: 'Superior treatment consists of dealing with an illness before it appears; mediocre treatment consists of curing an illness on the point of revealing itself; inferior treatment consists of curing the illness once it has manifested itself'.

As a fastidious physician, Sun also paid attention to the causes of illness, and his assessments in such matters were often insightful. He suggested, for example, that the origin of cholera needed to be sought in what people 'ate and drank' rather than in the influence of 'spirits'. He was interested in diseases caused by a deficiency of some kind such as beriberi; he treated nyctalopia (night-blindness) with goat or rabbit liver – it is known that this diminution of vision is due to a lack of vitamin A, with which liver is amply provided – or by prescribing decoctions of *Cassia obtusifolia*, whose seeds are still used in ophthalmology (notably in the case of glaucoma). Sun was also acquainted with the betel-nut (*Areca catechu*), which, as Jacques Roi points out, is used by the Chinese 'as a digestive, cough syrup, or an anthelminthic',[11] and he recommended its use in the treatment of tapeworm (taeniasis).

Sun was equally an enthusiastic advocate of maternal and infant care, insisting that vigilant attention be paid to the health of a pregnant woman. He advised future mothers to remain in a clean and calm environment and not to be nervous or apprehensive at the time of birth. (The same advice was intended for those in attendance on the mother.) If, after birth, the baby did not cry out, Sun proposed various procedures in the *Qianjin Yaofang* such as bathing the infant in warm water, blowing in its mouth and tapping on its body. He specified a fixed number of feeding-times and the amount of milk the baby was to consume. The wet-nurse, in Sun's opinion, had to be of gentle disposition and in good health.

Sun Simiao was to have a profound influence on future generations of Chinese and foreign physicians. One of them was the Japanese Nima Yasunori, who referred to Sun's work in his own treatise on prescriptions (*Yixinfang*, in the tenth century).

Su Jing and the *Newly-revised Materia Medica*

The *Xinxiu Bencao* (*Newly-revised Materia Medica*) was begun in 657 and completed in 659 under the direction of Su Jing, who had defended the project at the imperial court. It was the first Chinese (and world) official pharmacopoeia, preceding by eight or nine centuries the first official pharmacopoeia in the West, such as the *Nuovo Receptario*, which was published in Florence in 1498, or, especially, the *Pharmacopoeia of Nuremberg* of Valerius Cordus, which dates from 1546.[12] Introduced to Japan in 731 by Tanabe Fubito, the *Xinxiu Bencao* became a reference work for more than three centuries. It had a certain renown in Japan, judging by a

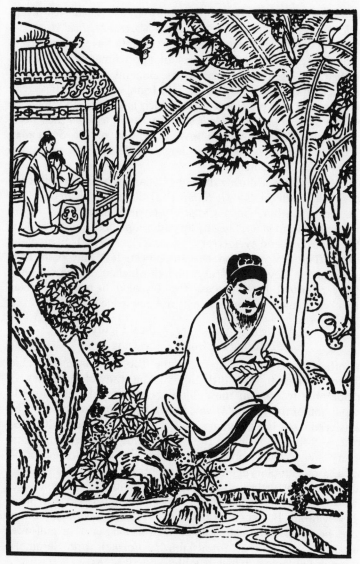

FIGURE 5.2   Sun Simiao. From *Zhongguo Gudai Yixuejia De Gushi* (Shanghai: Shaonian Ertong Chubanshe, 1979).

Japanese text of the early tenth century which noted that 'every physician needs Su Jing's *Newly-revised Materia Medica*'.[13]

The work, whose illustrations unfortunately have not survived, describes the therapeutic qualities of approximately 850 drugs classified by origin in nine categories; mineral, herbaceous plant, tree, quadruped, bird, insect and fish, fruit, vegetable and cereal. The editors of this pharmacopoeia, which later became known as the *Tang Bencao* (*Materia Medica of the Tang*), took as their point of departure Tao Hongjing's revised version of the *Shen'nong Bencaojing*. They revised and augmented the text with the description of 100 more drugs.

Chinese pharmacy during the Tang dynasty was further enriched with another text, the *Bencao Shiyi*. The title itself indicated the aim of the text's author, Chen Cangqi, who lived during the eighth century. The term *shiyi*, literally 'to gather up a lost object', alluded to the omissions and even errors in the works of Tao Hongjing and Su Jing. The *Bencao Shiyi* has since been lost, but both Tang Shiwei, in the eleventh century, and Li Shizhen, in the sixteenth century, refer to it. In the process, they revealed the range and detail of this 'supplement' to pharmaceutical knowledge of the time.

Wang Tao and Other Medical Figures during the Sui and the Tang

The official career taken up by Wang Tao, grandson of a chief minister, seemed to leave little time for the study of medicine. His considerable reading in the subject, however, culminated in the compilation of the *Waitai Miyao*, which he completed in 752. This magisterial work is a summary of all the fields explored by Chinese medicine from its origins to the eighth century: internal medicine, surgery, gynaecology, obstetrics, paediatrics, dermatology, orthopaedics, otorhinolaryngology and ophthalmology. Wang Tao's acumen was particularly evident in dealing with deficiency-induced illnesses; he recommended, for example, treating beriberi with plants rich in vitamin B1, such as plantain (*Plantago asiatica*). To cure goitre, he advised the use of algae such as sargasso, or gulf-weed (*Sargassum pallidum*; *Sargassum fusiforme*), and laminaria (*Laminaria japonica*), which is still used today.

Following in the footsteps of Sun Simiao, Wang Tao advocated the adoption of measures to ensure the protection of pregnant women, particularly at the time of birth. The *Waitai Miyao* and Sun Simiao's *Qianjin Yaofang* both occupy an important place in the history of gynaecology and obstetrics in China. Both works benefited from the favourable conditions during the Tang that contributed to the development of these two fields of medicine. The most noteworthy was doubtless the privileged position which women then occupied in Chinese society.[14] Sexuality, in fact, was one of the preoccupations of Chinese physicians at this time. Thus an entire section of the *Qianjin Yaofang* is devoted to sexual questions, or rather to 'the art of the bedroom' as described by Robert van Gulik in his book *Sexual Life in Ancient China*. The following extract from Sun Simiao's text is taken from van Gulik:

> A man must not engage in sexual intercourse merely to satisfy his lust. He must strive to control his sexual desire so as to be able to nurture his vital essence. He must not force his body to sexual extravagance in order to enjoy carnal pleasure, giving rein to his passion. On the contrary, a man must think of how the act will benefit his health, and thus keep himself free from disease.[15]

Other important figures of Chinese medicine during the Sui and Tang include Quan Yuanqi and Yang Shangshan, who helped promote a wider understanding of the *Huangdi Neijing*; the acupuncturist Zhen Quan (sixth and seventh centuries) and his brother Zhen Liyan, a herbalist who was particularly interested in parasitic diseases; Han Wenhai, who gained renown in Tibet; the dietician Meng Shen (c. 621–713), who specialised in macrobiotics; Wang Bing (c. 710–804), editor of the *Suwen* (*Essential Questions*); Gan Bozong, author of a collective biography on famous physicians, regrettably lost; Zan Yin, famous for his expertise in gynaecology and obstetrics; Li Xun, who specialised in medical substances of foreign origin; and Han Baosheng, whose *Materia Medica of Shu* (*Shu* is the classical name of Sichuan province, referred to by the eighth-century poet Li Bai in his lament 'Hard is the road in Shu') was later much appreciated by Tang Shenwei and Li Shizhen.

Notes

1. D. and V. Elisseeff, *La Civilisation de la Chine Classique*, op. cit., p 257.
2. Dominique Hoizey, *Li Po: Parmi les Nuages et les Pins*, op. cit.
3. Bai Juyi, *Poèmes*, translated by Dominique Hoizey (Reims: Albédo, 1985), p 7.
4. This refers to the unarmed tapeworm (*Taenia saginata*) that a person might contract by consuming uncooked or underdone beef (or buffalo meat) containing bladder-worm.
5. Bai Juyi, 'Le dragon de l'Etang noir', in *Poèmes*, op. cit., p 17.
6. Jacques Roi, *Traité des Plantes Médicinales Chinoises* (Paris: Paul Lechevalier, 1955), p 231.
7. Jean-Claude Dousset, *Histoire des Médicaments*, op. cit., p 57.
8. G. Tucci and W. Heissig, *Les Religions du Tibet et de la Mongolie* (Paris: Payot, 1973).

9. E. Brumpt and M. Neveu-Lemaire, *Travaux Pratiques de Parasit-ologie* (Paris: Masson et Cie, 1958), p 88, note: 'The sarcoptid is obtained by opening up the abcess and, with the point of a needle, extracting the white speck at the bottom of the groove. This white speck is in fact the female itch-mite.'

10. Catherine Despeux, op. cit., p 13.

11. Jacques Roi, *Traité des Plantes Médicinales Chinoises* op. cit., p 66.

12. See Jean-Claude Dousset, *Histoire des Médicaments,* op. cit., pp 93–4.

13. Cited in Yu Shenchu, *Zhongguo Yixue Jianshi*, op. cit., p 121.

14. See Ma Dazheng, 'Tangdai fuchan kexue gaikuang' (An overview of gynaecology and obstetrics during the Tang), *Zhonghua yishi zazhi* (*Chinese Journal of Medical History*), no 3 (1986).

15. Robert van Gulik, *Sexual Life in Ancient China* (Leiden, 1961), pp 193–4.

6

From the Northern to Southern Song, 960-1279

Barbarism and Civilisation

The fall of the Tang resulted in the disintegration of China. For the following fifty years, from 907-60, a series of short-lived dynasties was established in Kaifeng while the rest of the empire was divided up among independent kingdoms. The Song dynasty, founded in 960 by Zhao Guangyin, undertook to reunify the country. The momentum of such a campaign, however, was halted in the north by the Khitan, whose empire (known as the Liao) was sufficiently powerful to compel the Song dynasty to pay huge annual sums of money in order to guarantee peaceful relations. In the west, the Song confronted the menace of the Tibetans and then the Tanguts, with whom a costly peace treaty was signed in 1044. The barbarian threat finally came to fruition with the invasion of the Jurchen, founders of the Jin empire, who occupied north China and forced the Song to retreat to Hangzhou in the south, where the dynasty was to remain until the Mongol occupation of the late thirteenth century. The poetess Li Qingzhao (b. 1081) provides an echo of this national tragedy. Thinking of her motherland and of her forebears, she described her family's situation:

> For many years their descendants in the south
> Have led a wandering and homeless existence.[1]

During this period, traditionally divided between the Northern Song (960-1127) and Southern Song (1127-1279), China was buffeted by a series of reforms and counter-reforms. 'The most urgent need today is to acquire men of talent', declared Wang Anshi (1021-86). Wang's 'new laws' constituted 'the most radical political change China witnessed from the beginnings of the empire to the advent of communism'.[2] Wang's reforms in the fields of finance, the economy, army, administration and education aroused the opposition of conservatives such as the historian Sima Guang (1019–86), and were soon progressively abolished.

Economic expansion from the eleventh century to the thirteenth, sustained by the vigorous growth of agriculture, was facilitated by the emergence of an urban bourgeoisie whose extravagant lifestyle benefited handicraft production not only in ceramics but also, as Jacques Gernet emphasises, 'in all products affecting the comfort of daily life'.[3] The consequent commercial activity, both domestic and overseas, facilitated the development of river and maritime navigation, itself given an impetus by the closure of central Asian routes controlled by barbarian kingdoms. Moreover, navigation stimulated technological progress such as the use of the stern-rudder.

The availability of woodblock printing – the earliest printed text using this method dates from 868, although it was during the Song dynasty that Bi Sheng around 1040 invented moveable type – allowed for a greater diffusion of knowledge, particularly in the scientific domain. Numerous medical works were therefore published during this period, as well as treatises on the natural sciences and mathematics. Shen Gua (1031–95), mathematician, astronomer, physician and man of letters, dominated the world of science at this time, a time that also witnessed the revival of mathematics and new developments in geography and history. Especially noteworthy in history was the contribution of Sima Guang, whose *Zizhi Tongjian* (*General Mirror to Aid in Government*) had a lasting influence. Archaeology and epigraphy became fashionable. The *Collection of Inscriptions on Metal and Stone*, compiled by the erudite bibliophile and collector Zhao Mingcheng (1081–1129) with the collaboration of his wife, the poetess Li Qingzhao, testifies to this interest in antiquity.

China during the Song renewed its intellectual links with the philosophical tradition preceding the introduction of Buddhism. Confucius was 'rediscovered' through study of the Four Books (*The Analects, Mencius, The Great Learning* and *Doctrine of the Golden Mean*). The representatives of this 'new philosophy' – later known as neo-Confucianism – included Zhou Dunyi (1017–73), Zhang Zai (1020–77), who refocused on the notion of *qi* ('breath') as the sole reality, Cheng Hao (1032–85) and Cheng Yi (1033–1107), whose philosophy was based on the concept of *li*, the principle immanent in all things. The influence of their important successor, Zhu Xi (1130–1200), has been compared to that of Thomas Aquinas in the West.

The most significant figure in Chinese literature during this period was Su Dongpo (1037–1101), one of the outstanding poets of the Song dynasty along with Ouyang Xiu (1007–72), Mei Yaochen (1002–60), Li Qingzhao and Lu Yu (1125–1210). The Chinese sensibility was equally manifested in landscape painting.

A Publishing Boom

D. and V. Elisseeff note that Chinese printing 'seems to have benefited, even more than that of philosophical and literary works, the publication of scientific and technical treatises, whose appearance contributed to the improvement of daily life through the diffusion of a venerable tradition of theoretical and practical knowledge'.[4] It was with this aim that the Bureau for the Re-editing of Medical Books (*jiaozheng yishuju*) was created in 1057. This state institution aimed to collect, collate and verify all medical texts bequeathed by 1,000 years of history. In succession, the following works were published: *Suwen* (*Essential Questions*), the *Shanghanlun* (*On Cold-induced Maladies*) and *Jingui Yaolue* (*Summary from the Golden Chest*) by Zhang Zhongjing, the *Maijing* (*Pulse Classic*) by Wang Shuhe, the *Zhenjiu Jiayijing* (*ABC of Acupuncture*) by Huangfu Mi, the *Zhubing Yuanhoulun* (*Treatise on the Causes and Symptoms of Illnesses*) by Chao Yuanfang, and the *Qianjin Yaofang* (*Prescriptions*) by Sun Simiao. It was also under government patronage that a compilation of medical prescriptions was made at the end of the tenth century, known as the *Taiping Shenghuifang*; its principal author was Wang Huaiyin, a physician whose name is primarily associated with this work.

The *Taiping Shenghuifang* is more than a simple book of useful prescriptions (16,834 in all), since it embodied the essential medical knowledge of the time. At the beginning of the twelfth century, between 1107 and 1110, Chen Shiwen and Pei Zongyuan produced the *Hejijufang* (*Prescriptions from the Pharmacy of Harmonious Assistance*) which, in 1151, became known as the *Taiping Huimin Hejijufang*. Republished several times during the twelfth and thirteenth centuries, this work (as we know it today) lists 788 prescriptions with the appropriate information on how to prepare and use drugs. Finally, the *Shengji Zonglu* (*General Catalogue of Divine Assistance*), composed between 1111 and 1117, comprises a listing of 20,000 prescriptions and a medical summary of each illness, giving its causes, symptoms and respective cure.

The *Songshi* (*History of the Song*) includes a list of medical works published during the dynasty; the number and variety of such works testify to the flourishing state of Chinese medicine at this time. Most of the publications are concerned with internal medicine, such as the commentaries on the *Shanghanlun*, particularly those of Han Zhihe (*Shanghan Weizhi*: 'Hidden Meanings of the Shanghanlun') and Pang Anshi (*Shanghan Zongbinglun*: 'General Treatise on the Shanghanlun'), the *Sanyin Jiyi Bingzheng Fanglun* (*Treatise on Pathology based on the Theory of the Three Causes*) by Chen Yan, and the *Jishengfang* (*Prescriptions for Saving Life*) by Yan Yonghe. Other works listed in the catalogue deal with those affecting children, such as Qian Yi's *Xiao'er Yaozheng Zhijue* (*The Appropriate Way of Recognising and Treating Infant Maladies*) and Chen Wenzhong's *Xiao'er Bingyuan Fanglun* (*Treatise on the Origin of Infant Maladies*), gynaecology and obstetrics, surgery, such as Chen Ziming's *Waike Jingyao* (*Essentials of Surgery*), acupuncture and moxibustion, pulsing and hygiene.

'Materia medica' (works on herbal medicine) thrived from the beginning of the dynasty with the compilation of the *Kaibao Bencao* (*Herbal Medicine of the Kaobao Era*) in 973; it was revised one year later under the title *Kaibao Chongding Bencao* (*Revised Herbal Medicine of the Kaibao Era*). In 1057, Su Song, Zhang Yuxi and others began the compilation of the *Jiayou Buzhu Bencao* (*Complete and Annotated Materia Medica of the Jiayou Era*); it was published in 1061. The same Su Song also wrote the *Tujing Bencao* (*Illustrated Materia Medica*), which will be discussed later. At the end of the eleventh century, Tang Shenwei compiled the *Zhenglei Bencao* (*Classified Materia Medica*), which was revised by Ai Sheng in 1108 and became the official *Daguan Bencao* (*Materia Medica of the Daguan Era*). A new version of this work, entitled the *Zhenghe Bencao* (*Materia Medica of the Zhenghe Era*), was begun in 1116 by Cao Xiaozhong. In the same year, Kou Zongshi published the *Bencao Yanyi*.

Chinese medicine during the Song dynasty also had its forensic experts and historians, and they too published their work. Thus an important treatise on forensic medicine, the *Xiyuan Jilu* by Song Ci, appeared in 1247. It was preceded by the earliest text on the history of Chinese medicine in existence today, the *Yishou* by Zhang Gao, which dates from 1189.

The Reform of Medical Studies, Autopsies Carried Out on Executed Prisoners, and the Creation of Forensic Medicine

The interest in medicine shown by the Song authorities led not only to official support for the publication of general medical works but also to a new surge in medical studies. The reforms launched by Wang Anshi during the eleventh century in the educational domain, particularly in connection with the curriculum and examination system, were applied to medical instruction. This last came under the jurisdiction of the Imperial Bureau of Medicine (*Taiyiju*), which supervised the medical schools gradually established in each prefecture during the eleventh and twelfth centuries. Medical studies were reorganised on the pattern of the civil service examination system, that is three levels of attainment were created based on monthly and annual examinations. Each examination had three grades: 'excellent', 'fair' and 'poor'. The curriculum comprised thirteen disciplines grouped under three sections: internal medicine, acupuncture and 'illnesses of the skin' (*yang*). The last included dermatology and traumatology, while otorhinolaryngology and ophthalmology came under the acupuncture section, and paediatrics was assigned to the internal medicine section. Instruction in medical theory primarily relied on the *Suwen* (*Essential Questions*), the *Nanjing* (*Classic of Difficult Problems*), the *Zhubing Yuanhoulun* (*Treatise on the Causes and Symptoms of Illnesses*), the *Qianjin Yaofang* (*Prescriptions of the Thousand Ounces of Gold*) and the *Buzhu Bencao* (*Complete and Annotated Materia Medica*). The *Maijing* (*Pulse Classic*) and *Shanghanlun* (*On Cold-induced Maladies*) completed the curriculum for those studying internal medicine, and the *Zhenjiu Jiayijing* (*ABC of Acupuncture*) for those in the acupuncture section. Overall, therefore, medical instruction adhered closely to the tradition bequeathed by the 'fathers of Chinese medicine', from Qin Yueren to Sun Simiao. Later, new theories such as that of the 'three causes', expounded by Chen Yan at the end of the twelfth century, would be added to the curriculum.

Medical studies also benefited from a greater familiarity with anatomy due to the practice of dissection. The first known dissection to be carried out, recounted in the *Qianhanshu* (*History of the Former Han*), dates from the beginning of the Christian era, but during the Song dynasty anatomical plates began to be used. First there were those drawn up during the years 1041–8, outlining the anatomy of a certain Ou Xifan, an executed bandit. Then, at the beginning of the twelfth century, there appeared the *Cunzhentu*, which brought together illustrations of the dissections ordered by the prefect of Suzhou, Li Yixing, to be carried out on the corpses of executed prisoners. The illustrator was the physician and poet, Yang Jie (1068–1140).

One of the most notable medical developments during the Song was the establishment of forensic medicine with the publication of the *Xiyuan Jilu* by Song Ci (1186–1249). It was to serve as a model for numerous works in this field until the end of the nineteenth century. The *Xiyuan Jilu* contains recommendations on how to carry out autopsies, but with its observations concerning physiology, histology, pathology, pharmacology and toxicology the work has enormous significance for the history of medicine in China.

The use of poison attracts special attention in the *Xiyuan Jilu*. The famous novel *Jin Ping Mei* (*Golden Lotus*), the action of which takes place towards the end of the Northern Song, recounts how the supervisor of dissections, He Jiu, allows himself to be bribed and attributes the death of Wu the Elder to natural causes when evidence shows that he had in fact been poisoned:

> One noticed immediately how much suffering the man had endured because of his bluish nails, purple lips, waxy complexion and protruding eyes. The two assistants protested: 'How is it that even his face is purple, that his lips bear the trace of teeth-marks and that blood is dripping from his mouth?' 'Be quiet, and no more stupid remarks', interrupted He Jiu. 'With the warm weather these last few days, how can you not expect that the corpse would show some deterioration?' . . . Dealing with the case forthwith, He Jiu authorised the burial without any further investigation.[5]

How was poisoning recognised? 'A person who has died of poison', explains the *Xiyuan Jilu*, 'has a wide-open mouth and eyes, a greenish or dark violet complexion, purple lips, completely blue fingernails and toenails, and blood trickling from the mouth, eyes, ears and nose'. To confirm such a prognosis, the *Xiyuan Jilu* suggests inserting a silver needle, scrubbed and washed in soapy water, into the mouth of the deceased. Shortly afterwards, the needle should be extracted and its blackish colour will be evident. Attempts to scrub and wash the needle in soapy water will be to no avail.[6] An entire section of the *Xiyuan Jilu* is devoted to emergency care, particularly in poisoning cases.

A New Approach to Aetiology: The Theory of the 'Three Causes'

The theory of the 'three causes' (*sanyin*), mentioned earlier, was first propounded by a physician of the twelfth century, Chen Yan. The originality of his most important work, a treatise on pathology entitled *Sanyin Jiyi Bingzheng*, lay in its new approach to aetiology. According to Chen Yan, there were three kinds of pathogenic agents: endogenous, exogenous, and those neither one nor the other. The seven endogenous agents were joy (*xi*), anger (*nu*), vexation (*you*), sadness (*si*), distress (*bei*), fear (*kong*) and fright (*jing*). The six exogenous agents were wind (*feng*), cold (*han*), heat (*shu*), humidity (*shi*), drought (*zao*) and fire (*huo*). The third kind of agent referred in fact to those exogenous agents not specifically included in the second category, and included all types of chance mishaps from snake-bites to wounds inflicted by knives or swords.

Traditional Chinese medicine has preserved this concept of endogenous and exogenous agents. The authors of *Zhongyixue Jichu (Essential Book of Chinese Medicine)* note that endogenous agents primarily refer to the 'seven feelings' (*qing*) which 'can lead to an imbalance between the *yin* and *yang* in the body, between vital energy (*qi*) and the blood, and to the irregular functioning of the meridians (*jingluo*) and the *zang* and *fu* organs, all of which give rise to illness'.[7] Psychic influences on the mind, for example, might provoke palpitations, insomnia and loss of memory. The six exogenous factors are none other than the influence of the seasons, to which, according to the *Suwen* section of the *Huangdi Neijing*, man must adapt. Thus in spring, when 'heaven and earth together produce life', it is incumbent upon man to pay particular attention to his health; 'to go against the tide will bring harm to the liver',[8] the *zang* organ associated with spring. The *Zhongyixue Jichu (Essential Book of Chinese Medicine)* says precisely this: 'The wind, cold, heat, humidity, drought and fire are the six climatic variations of nature, the "six influences"'. However, when the human body, due to a reduced capacity for resistance, 'cannot adapt to these climatic changes, or when the abnormal weather change outstrips the body's capacity to adapt, the six influences then become pathogenic factors'.[9] In this situation, the 'influences' (*qi*) are referred to as 'excesses' (*yin*) that can cause illness. Like Chen Yan, Chinese medical tradition observes a third category of pathogenic factors, which include intemperance, fatigue, traumatism and even the presence of parasites in the body.

The First Measures against Smallpox

The Song dynasty witnessed the development of public welfare in the urban areas with the opening of dispensaries, hospitals and orphanages. Urbanisation obliged the authorities to make special arrangements for public hygiene; in Hangzhou, for example, during the Southern Song, road-sweepers and night-soil collectors were a daily presence. Evidence also points to the use of spittoons. The most outstanding preventive measure, however, would be the resort to anti-smallpox vaccinations, at least if there were incontestable evidence of such a practice at this particular time. The *Niudou Xinshu (New Work on Anti-Smallpox Vaccine)*, published in 1884, dates the beginnings of vaccination to the years 713–41, during which a certain person by the name of Zhao used for the first time the method of inoculating in the nostril of a patient a small amount of variolous pustules. Another text, the *Douzhen Dinglun* (*Established Principles of Smallpox*), which dates from 1713, recounts that in the eleventh century, during the reign of Emperor Renzong, a recluse from Mount Emei inoculated the son of prime minister Wang Dan against smallpox. The opinion expressed by Yu Maokun in his *Douke Jinjing Fujijie* (*Explanations of Smallpox*), published in 1727, is much more credible. According to Yu, anti-smallpox vaccinations date from the years 1567–72, although it was not until the publication of *Zhangshi Yitong* (*Medical Compendium of Master Zhang*) in 1695 and *Yizong Jinjian* (*Golden Mirror of Medicine*) in 1742 that a detailed description of vaccination methods used in China to combat smallpox was given. Whatever the case, Chinese physicians most certainly preceded Jenner in the use of vaccinations; Voltaire was not the last to acknowledge China's pioneering role:

> I learn that the Chinese have resorted to vaccination for the last hundred years; this is a significant precedent to be emulated, originating in a country that passes for the wisest and best-governed in the world. It is true that the Chinese go about it in a different way; they do not make any incision but rather insert the smallpox virus through the nose like snuff tobacco. This method is more agreeable, but in any case serves the same purpose, confirming that if inoculation had been practised in France, thousands of lives would have been saved.[10]

Paediatricians and Gynaecologists

The authors of *Zhongguo Yixueshi* (*A History of Chinese Medicine*) note that 'during the Song and Yuan dynasties, paediatrics became a specialised and independent branch of medicine, obtaining significant results'.[11] The most important figure in the field was without doubt Qian Yi (1035–1117). Orphaned at an early age, Qian Yi was taken in by his uncle, who taught him medicine. He devoted forty years of his life to the treatment of children; Qian Yi's diagnoses were recorded by his disciple Yan Xiaozhong in the *Xiao'er Yaozheng Zhijue* (*The Appropriate Way of Recognising and Treating Infant Maladies*). This work deals entirely with infant medicine, considered under its physiological, pathological and therapeutic aspects. Certain medications have been preserved to the present, such as the decoction of *Cimicifuga foetida* and *Pueraria lobata* prescribed by Qian Yi especially to treat smallpox and which traditional Chinese medicine continues to recommend for the treatment of measles. Moreover, Qian Yi contributed to a better understanding of eruptive fevers such as smallpox, chickenpox and measles, in terms both of symptomatology and of therapy.

Smallpox, which was probably the cause for a high infant mortality rate, stimulated the development of paediatrics as a vocation, and those who took up the calling all devoted time to the disease. One such paediatrician was Dong Ji, whose *Xiao'er Banzhen Beiji Fanglun* (dating from 1093) was the first published work in China on smallpox. Nearly 150 years later, in 1241, there appeared a treatise by Chen Wenzhong, the *Xiao'er Douzhen Fanglun*, which was a study of smallpox among children. Chen Wenzhong also wrote a work on paediatrics, the *Xiao'er Bingyuan Fanglun* (*Treatise on the Origins of Infant Maladies*), in which he advised especially on ways to protect children's health. He recommended, for example, that children be given warm food and drink, should consume liquids as often as possible, and should avoid any dietary excess. The cause of paediatrics during the Song dynasty was served by other physicians such as Liu Fang (c. 1080–1150), whose *Youyou Xinshu* (*New Work on Children*) appeared in 1132; it encompassed the sum of contemporary medical knowledge concerning infant illnesses. Several years later, in 1156, the Imperial Bureau of Medicine published the *Xiao'er Weisheng Zongwei Lunfang*, one of the most important treatises on paediatrics during the Song along with Qian Yi' *Xiao'er Yaozheng Zhijue* and Liu Fang's *Youyou Xinshu*. This list of paediatric works would not be complete without mention of the *Renzhai Zhizhi Xiao'er Fanglun*, an inventory of childhood illnesses drawn up by Yang Shiying (alias Renzhai) in the 1260s.

The Song period also witnessed a fruitful development in the fields of gynaecology and obstetrics, which were dominated by two names – those of Chen Ziming and Zhu Duanzhong. The earliest work on gynaecology and obstetrics was the *Chanbao* (literally: 'Treasure of Childbirth'), written by a Tang dynasty physician, Zan Yin, during the years 852–6. He was followed in this field by Guo Jizhong, who wrote a treatise on obstetrics in the twelfth century, the *Chanyu Baoqingji*.

Gynaecology and obstetrics at this time was beginning to take on the hallmarks of an independent branch of medicine. Specialised works in the field were published, including the *Furen Daquan Liangfang* by Chen Ziming (c. 1190–1270). This work, dating from 1237, deals with various gynaecological problems associated with menstruation, pregnancy and childbirth. How was pregnancy diagnosed at this time? First of all, by an interruption of menstruation, but to be absolutely sure Chen Ziming prescribed a decoction of *chuanxiong* (*Ligusticum wallichii*), whose effect was to induce uterine contractions. Chen's concern to protect the foetus and, if possible, to prevent miscarriage or to delay premature birth prompted him to prohibit the consumption of certain herbal drugs such as the root of the *Achyranthes bidentata*, known as an emmenagogue (agent that increases or renews menstrual discharge), croton, or even the plant known as white hellebore (*Veratrum nigrum*), which has emetic properties and is still advised against today for pregnant women.[12] Besides vomiting, other ailments affecting pregnant women such as puerperal eclampsia (convulsions) were described by Chen Ziming. A whole chapter of his book is devoted to cases of difficult childbirth. Several examples of dystocia (painful childbirth) are described: shoulder-delivery, face-delivery and breech-delivery. The other important name in the field of gynaecology and obstetrics is that of Zhu Duanzhang, whose treatise on obstetrics, the *Weisheng Jiabao Chanke Beiyao*, dates from 1184. He was preceded by Yang Zijian who, at the end of the eleventh century, wrote the *Shichanlun*, the earliest text in the history of Chinese medicine that mentions the version method, an operation of manually turning the child so as to facilitate delivery.

The Great Leap Forward in Acupuncture

A bronze man contributed to the development of acupuncture from the eleventh century onwards. The creator of this figure, Wang Weiyi (c. 987–1067), had the idea of casting two statues in bronze representing a man from the front and from behind. On these statues were engraved the 657 acupuncture points. One can imagine the paedagogical significance of such objects. At the same time, Wang Weiyi compiled his celebrated *Tongren Shuxue Zhen Jiu Tujing* (*Illustrated Manual of the Bronze Man Showing Acupuncture and Moxibustion Points*). Moreover, the text of this work was engraved on two stone steles more than two metres high and seven metres in width, and were erected at Kaifeng, capital of the Northern Song dynasty, for public benefit.

The *Songshi* (*History of the Song*) recounts that Emperor Renzong, who fell ill in 1034, was cured successfully through acupuncture. This helped to popularise a therapeutic method that became the forte of specialised physicians such as Wang Zhizhong during the Southern Song dynasty. Wang was the author of a description of acupuncture and moxibustion, published in 1220, the *Zhenjiu Zishengjing*. Moxibustion itself was the subject of a treatise published in 1226, the *Beiji Jiufa*. The author, Wen-ren Qinian, referred to various cases of acute infection, such as toothache, that could be cured through cauterisation.

Adepts of the *Shanghanlun*, Experts on Pulsing, and
Remedies for All Afflictions from a Chill to Breast Cancer

If one had to summarise in a few lines the history of Chinese
medicine during the Song, one might simply refer to the names of
Yang Jie (anatomy), Chen Yan (aetiology), Qian Yi and Chen
Wenzhong (paediatrics), Chen Ziming and Zhu Duanzhang
(gynaecology and obstetrics), Wang Weiyi (acupuncture) and Song
Ci (forensic medicine), who all certainly contributed to the
development of their particular specialised fields. However,
numerous other practitioners helped in the progress of Chinese
medicine. One might begin with those who wrote commentaries on
the *Shanghanlun*, the classic of Chinese medicine that dealt with
illnesses subsumed under the category of *shanghan*. Such illnesses,
in the absence of a precise definition, might be characterised as a
feverish state brought on by an external agent.

Pang Anshi was one of these commentators. Around 1100, he
wrote the *Shanghan Zongbinglun* (*General Treatise on Shanghan
Illnesses*). A reading of Pang's treatise reveals that the therapeutic
methods recommended by Zhang Zhongjing had hardly changed:
sweating (sudation), induced vomiting and purging remained the
principal cures of *shanghan* illnesses. Such methods were
emphasised by other physicians such as Zhu Gong, Han Zhihe and
Qian Wenli. Zhu Gong (born in the eleventh century) spent ten
years of his life studying the *Shanghanlun*; the fruits of his labours
culminated in 1107 with the *Nanyang Huorenshu*, a work whose
alternative title, *Shanghan Baiwen* (*100 Questions on Shanghan
Illnesses*), indicates the special approach of its theoretical section,
written in the form of questions and answers. In addition, the work
has particular interest for its description of the remedies prescribed
by the *Shanghanlun*, making it as significant a text as the
Shanghanlun itself. Han Zhihe wrote *Shanghan Weizhi* (*Hidden
Meanings of Shanghan Illnesses*) at the end of the twelfth century.
Finally, there appeared in 1162 the *Shanghan Baiwenge* (*100
Questions in Song on Shanghan Illnesses*). The author, Qian Wenli,
had the novel idea of using rhymed verse in order to assist
memorisation.

This enthusiasm for the *Shanghanlun* was shared by physicians
of the Jin dynasty (1115–1234), established in Kaifeng. The
commentary by Cheng Wuji (born between 1056 and 1067) is
particularly well-known. Entitled the *Zhujie Shanghanlun*, it is an
annotated edition of the *Shanghanlun* dating from 1144. Cheng
Wuji was also the author of *A Concise Description of Shanghan
Illnesses*.

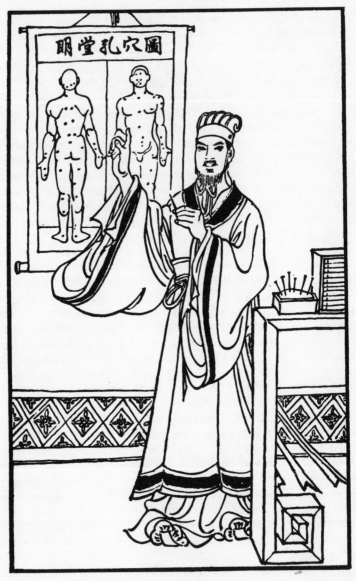

FIGURE 6.1   Wang Weiyi. From *Zhongguo Gudai Yixuejia De Gushi*
(Shanghai: Shaonian Ertong Chubanshe, 1979).

For the physician of the eleventh and twelfth centuries, whether he was a follower of the *shanghan* school or not, taking the pulse was fundamental in arriving at a diagnosis. The key reference work remained Wang Shuhe's *Maijing* (*Pulse Classic*) which, moreover, constituted part of the curriculum laid down by the Imperial Bureau of Medicine. Cui Jiayan relied on the *Maijing*, as well as on the *Maijue* (*Principles of the Pulse*) by Gao Yangsheng, in writing the *Cuishi Maijue* (*Principles of the Pulse by Master Cui*) at the end of the twelfth century, which was composed in four-character verse. Li Shizhen appended the text in his own 1564 treatise on pulsing, the *Binhu Maixue* (*Binhu's Study of the Pulse*). Undoubtedly the most important figure of Chinese pulsing during the Song dynasty was Shi Fa, author in 1241 of the *Chabing Zhinan* (*A Guide for the Examination of Illness*), in which taking the pulse occupies a central role. Based on an examination of his own pulse, Shi Fa drew up a diagram outlining its workings six centuries before the invention of the sphygmograph (instrument recording movements of the pulse) by Marey in 1860.

The next step after diagnosis was treatment. Prescription books were not lacking. In addition to those mentioned at the beginning of this chapter (*Taiping Shenghuifang, Taiping Huimin Hejijufang, Shengji Zonglu*), published on the authorisation of the state, reference should also be made to more than a dozen other titles. Chief among these was the *Jishengfang* (*Prescriptions for Saving Life*), completed by Yan Yonghe (c. 1200–67) in 1253. Some of the prescriptions included in this work are still used today, such as the tonic decoction known as *gui pi tang*.[13] Other significant contributions include *Su Shen Liangfang* (*Efficacious Prescriptions of Su and Shen*), by Su Shi (Su Dongpo), the poet, and Shen Gua, the renowned scholar of science during the Northern Song; and the *Puji Benshifang* (*Effective Prescriptions for the Relief of All*) by Xu Shiwei (1080–1154?), two-thirds of whose 366 prescriptions recommend the use of pills, powders, ointments, medical alcohol, rice porridge, acupuncture and moxibustion, and massage. Decoctions are only mentioned in a third of the prescriptions; they include the well-known ones from the *Shanghanlun* (*Ephedra sinica, Cinnamomum cassia* and *Pueraria lobata*), a text that particularly fascinated Xu Shiwei and to which he devoted several works. Mention might also be made of the *Wangshi Bojifang* (*Master Wang's Prescriptions For the Help of All*) by Wang Gun in 1247, a collection of prescriptions compiled by the paediatrician Dong Ji in 1086 for the benefit of travellers, the *Lüshe Beiyao Fang* (*Emergency Prescriptions for Those Staying at Inns*), Shi Kan's collection compiled around 1101 known as the *Shi Zaizhi Fang* (*Prescriptions of Shi Zaizhi*) and, finally, the collections of Wang Kuang (1125), Yang Tan (1178), Wu Yankui (1180) and Zhu Zuo (1265).

Of all the diseases treated in this period, one in particular merits particular attention – cancer. Significantly, it was in an anonymous work of the twelfth century, the *Weiji Baoshu* (*Precious Book for Protection and Relief*), that the character for cancer, *ai*, appeared for the first time. The *Weiji Baoshu* describes the case of a woman in her forties affected by breast cancer and who died after three years of treatment. In 1264, Yang Shiying, already mentioned in his role as a paediatrician, gave a description of cancer in the *Renzhai Zhizhi Fanglun* as 'poisoned roots that are deeply hidden and which bore into and penetrate the interior'. Tumours and abscesses of all kinds, a wide variety of inflammations, furunculosis and other skin disorders were all treated in the appropriate manner, such as drainage of the pus through acupuncture or cauterisation, with the patient ultimately being given fortifying drugs. Certain disorders, which up until now have been dealt with by minor surgery, were treated exclusively with the aid of oral drugs; this is shown in such works as the *Shengji Zonglu* (in which arsenic is recommended for the treatment of haemorrhoids), the *Jiyan Beijufang* (1196) by Li Xun, and the *Waike Jingyao* (*Essentials of Surgery*) written in 1263 by Chen Ziming, one of the most important gynaecologists of the Song dynasty.

The Pharmaceutical Renaissance

The relations which China enjoyed between the tenth and twelfth centuries with its neighbours (Korea, Japan and South-east Asia), as well as with the contemporary Arab world, facilitated mutual exchanges in the fields of medicine and pharmacy. Among the items of tribute offered by various states to the Chinese emperor, it was not uncommon to find mineral, vegetable and animal products that were to be used in the manufacture of medicine. The *Songshi* (*History of the Song*) gives several examples, but the most striking evidence of this foreign contribution to Chinese medicine is provided by the statues erected in front of the several imperial tombs of the Northern Song.[14] Among the statues in front of the tomb of Emperor Zhenzong (998–1022) is one that represents a foreign envoy carrying a rhinoceros horn. According to the *Songshi*, Jiaozhi (present-day Vietnam) offered tribute of rhinoceros horns in 998 and 1010. The earliest reference to rhinoceros horns, which are used in Chinese pharmacy, is found in the *Shen'nong Bencaojing*. A sculpture in front of the tomb of Emperor Taizong (976–97) depicts an offering of elephant tusks by an ambassador who most probably comes from an Indonesian kingdom that supplied China with ivory at this time. Another envoy holds a bottle of rose-water, while a third figure presents a goblet of pearls. The use of pearls in Chinese pharmacy is mentioned for the first time in the *Kaibao Chongding Bencao* (*Revised Materia Medica of the Kaibao Era*), which dates from 974. The celebrated Song dynasty book of prescriptions, the *Hejijufang* (abbreviated title of the *Taiping Huimin Hejijufang*), prescribes a treatment using pearl dust for the cure of a sore throat, while the *Shengji Zonglu* (which dates from the beginning of the twelfth century) recommends a powder and pills made up from crushed pearls.[15]

Finally, two other statues are relevant for the history of Chinese pharmacy. One is situated in front of the tomb of Emperor Renzong (1023–63), and the other in front of that of Emperor Zhezong (1086–1100). The former depicts someone carrying a tray of coral and the latter an elephant holding a melon in its trunk. Coral is mentioned in connection with several drugs described in the *Xinxiu Bencao* (*Newly-revised Materia Medica*) of Su Jing. During the Song period, coral is described in the Bencao Yanyi and the *Taiping Shenghuifang* as an ophthalmic drug.[16] The sweet melon (*tiangua, Cucumis melo*) already had a long pharmaceutical history, since it is included among the superior drugs described in the *Shen'nong Bencaojing.*

Mention has been made earlier of the burgeoning output of medical and pharmaceutical works during the Song dynasty, among which were several materia medica. Heir to the materia medica compiled during the preceding Tang dynasty, the *Kaibao Bencao* (983 drugs) and the *Jiayou Bencao* (1,082 drugs) were part of a long series of such works, supplemented in 1061 by Su Song's *Zhenglei Bencao* (*Classified Materia Medica*). Su Song (1017–1101) collaborated with Zhang Yuxi, Lin Yi and Gao Baoheng in the revision of materia medica then in use. Their endeavours culminated in 1061 with the *Jiayou Buzhu Shen'nong Bencaojing* (*Completed and Annotated Classic of Herbal Medicine of the Jiayou Era*), abbreviated to *Jiayou Bencao*. The text itself is lost, but its contents appeared in various later works, in particular Tang Shenwei's *Zhenglei Bencao*. Su Song at this time also produced the *Tujing Bencao*, which was both to inspire Tang Shenwei several years later and to find an echo in Li Shizhen's magisterial work of the sixteenth century, the *Bencao Gangmu*.

Along with Su Song, Tang Shenwei (c. 1056–93) dominated the field of herbal medicine, and his *Zhenglei Bencao* was to remain the

model for the next 500 years. There were several versions of the
work, including one revised and amended by Ai Sheng in 1108
(*Materia Medica of the Daguan Era*), and another by Cao Xiaozhong
in 1116 (*Materia Medica of the Zhenglei Era*). Other versions were
published in 1159 and 1249. Tang Shenwei compiled his materia
medica about 1108, carrying on the work of his predecessor, Su
Song, who wrote the *Tujing Bencao*. Tang's materia medica was
also illustrated, and it contained descriptions of certain drugs for
the first time in the history of Chinese herbal medicine. The edition
of 1249 lists 1,746 drugs, while the original edition only lists 1,558
(of which only 476 were not mentioned in previous works on herbal
medicine). Herbal medicine, in full bloom at this time, was the
subject of various other publications, including the *Bencao Yanyi*
(*Development of Herbal Medicine*) by Kou Zongshi in 1116.

Notes

1. Li Qingzhao, *OEuvres Poétiques Complètes*, translated by Liang
   Paitchin (Paris: Gallimard, 1977), p 129.
2. D. and V. Elisseeff, *La Civilisation de la Chine Classique*, op.
   cit., pp 407–8.
3. Jacques Gernet, *A History of Chinese Civilization*, op. cit., p 322.
4. D. and V. Elisseeff, *La Civilisation de la Chine Classique*, op.
   cit., p 461.
5. *Jin Ping Mei* (*Golden Lotus*), translated by André Lévy (Paris:
   Gallimard, 1985), p 118.
6. Based on the extracts of the *Xiyuan Jilu* cited by Yu Shenchu in
   Zhongguo Yixue Jianshi, op. cit., p 162. I have translated the
   expression *zaojiu shui* as 'soapy water'. Literally it means 'water
   of the gleditschia' (*Gleditschia sinensis*), a tree whose pods contain
   saponins.
7. *Zhongyixue Jichu* (*Essential Book of Chinese Medicine*) (Beijing:
   Renmin Weisheng Chubanshe, 1984), p 41.
8. From the translation of the *Suwen* by Claude Larre and Elisabeth
   Rochat de La Vallée, *Assaisonner les Esprits* (Paris: Institut
   Ricci, 1985), p 15.
9. *Zhongyixue Jichu*, op. cit., p 34.
10. Voltaire, 'Onzième Lettres philosophique: Sur l'insertion de la
    petite vérole', in *Lettres Philosophiques* (Paris: Garnier-Flammarion,
    1964).
11. *Zhongguo Yixueshi* (Shanghai: Shanghai Kexue Jishu Chubanshe,
    1984), p 69.
12. *Quanguo Zhongcaoyao Huibian* (Beijing: Renmin Jishu Chubanshe,
    1975, 1983), vol. 1, p 931: 'This plant is toxic; it needs to be used
    carefully, while pregnant women are advised not to take it'. The
    rhizome of the *Veratrum nigrum* is rich in extremely toxic steroid
    alkaloids. It also has parasitical properties. As for the *Achyranthes
    bidentata*, research done in 1980 has revealed the uterotonic
    effect of the saponin (oleic acid) extracted from the plant. See
    Yip, Fung, Kong, Akiyama and Sankawa, 'Uterotonic Activity of

Achyranthes bidentata Saponins', Fourth Asian Symposium on Medicinal Plants and Spices, Bangkok, 15–19 September 1980.

13. *Zhongyixue Jichu,* op. cit., p 249.

14. These tombs are located in Gong district (Gong xian), Henan province, less than 100 kilometres to the west of Zhengzhou. See 'Beisong huangling zhongyao shike diaocha baogao' (Report on the research into the sculptures of Chinese drugs at the Northern Song Imperial tombs), *Zhonghua Yishi Zazhi*, no 4 (1986), pp 256–9.

15. Current research is being carried out on two kinds of pearl-bearing oysters: *Pteria martensii* and *Pteria margaritifera.* Their pearls are used in medicine in the form of powder or pills.

16. Coral (*Corallium*) is still being used today in Chinese ophthalmology, especially for the treatment of leucoma.

7

The Jin,
1115–1234,
and Yuan,
1279–1368

From the Jin Empire to the Mongol Occupation

In 1115, the Jurchen, non-Chinese tribes from the present-day northern province of Heilongjiang, established the Jin empire. Its hegemonic ambitions prompted an attack on the Song, forcing the latter to retreat southwards from the Yellow River basin to Jiangnan (i.e. south of the Yangzi). During the thirteenth century, the Mongols rose to prominence, overthrowing the Jin in 1234 and then, in 1279, the Southern Song. The new Mongol dynasty, which adopted the Chinese name of Yuan, held sway throughout China and instituted a system whose major feature, as Jacques Gernet observes, was the clear differentiation among Mongols, Chinese and other ethnic groups. Such differentiation went as far as prohibiting marriage between the ethnic groups.[1] Mongol oppression bore heavily on the peasantry, which was burdened with forced labour and taxes. The peasantry were not the only ones to suffer, however, since the policies carried out by the Yuan rulers and their advisers led to the impoverishment of Chinese society as a whole. The century of Mongol rule, moreover, was marked by a series of popular revolts led by secret societies or Buddhist-inspired millenarian movements.

On the other hand, Mongol expansion benefited merchants from Central Asia, the Middle East, or even elsewhere, such as the Polo family from Europe. The family's most famous member, Marco Polo (1254–1324), was entrusted with confidential missions by the emperor Kubilai Khan. Christianity also attempted to gain a foothold in China, notably in the person of John of Montecorvino (1247–1328), who became archbishop of Khanbalik, present-day Beijing. Islamic influence, too, penetrated the Chinese world during the era of Mongol rule. The Chinese, for their part, including a Daoist

90

monk, Qiu Chuji (of whom more will be said later), travelled to foreign lands, enriching other cultures with new ideas, particularly in the technological domain.

Science and technology, dominated by the mathematicians Guo Shoujing (1231–1316), who used his talents in astronomy and hydrography, and Zhu Shijie, the author of renowned treatises on mathematics around 1300, benefited from the willing support provided by the Mongol authorities. The Mongol rulers, however, in the process of imposing a strictly-regulated system of medical practice, banned the use of certain toxic drugs. In 1268, the sale of aconite[2] and arsenic was forbidden. In a play entitled *Black Whirlwind Yields a Double Retribution* (the Yuan period was a golden age of Chinese theatre), the following dialogue takes place:

> Li (*aside*):   I've brought with me a sleeping potion made up of
>   arsenic and oil of croton, which I shall mix in with
>   the food. When he's eaten he'll sleep until tomorrow
>   at least. (To the gaoler.) Old man, go on, eat.
> Gaoler: Okay, give me the dish. (He blows.)
> Li: Old man, why are you blowing?
> Gaoler: I'm blowing on the arsenic and oil of croton. (He
>   eats.) Ah! this is a famous dish. You've spiced it in
>   a funny way, though, you scoundrel. Anyway, I've
>   scoffed it all. (He then falls in a heap.)
> Li: Come on gaoler, stand up! Good, he's incapable of
>   moving, now we shall be left alone until tomorrow.
>   I can get on with freeing my brother.[3]

Fear of poisoning was often invoked as justification for the regulation of drug-use, which was reinforced by other draconian measures. From 1272, anyone buying or selling prohibited drugs was liable to be punished with death. Finally, in 1311, a new list of banned drugs was drawn up, which included (in addition to those mentioned above) laurel, euphorbia and henbane. At the same time, the medical profession itself was strictly supervised in order to weed out fraudsters.

The world of Chinese medicine (one should also note the existence of Mongol medical practitioners, who were particularly adept in the art of setting fractures) during the Jin and Yuan dynasties was one of differing schools, with physicians following their own respective masters and teachings, and whose medical concepts (doctrinal and therapeutic) either intermingled or stood in mutual opposition. In order to understand these debates, it is useful to recall certain essential notions of Chinese medicine and pharmacy.

Symptoms and Drugs

Chinese symptomatology relied on various ways of investigating the manifestation of a disease, all based on the acceptance of the eight guiding principles (*bagang, ba*, 'eight'; *gang*, 'the principal string of a net', 'principle'): those of external (*biao*) and internal (*li*), cold (*han*) and hot (*re*), depletion (*xu*) and excess (*shi*), *yin* and *yang*. The tendency was to equate each of these principles with a particular syndrome, that is to say 'a number of symptoms which collectively indicate an often abnormal condition of the body or mind'. The syndrome associated with the external principle was distinguished (*bian*: 'to distinguish') by the following signs: fever, headache, furry tongue and prominent pulse, symptoms that prompted the physician to recommend sweating the patient. The syndrome associated with the internal principle affected the *zang* and *fu* organs. The syndrome associated with the cold principle was revealed by a pale complexion, among other clinical signs, while that associated with the hot principle was characterised by fever, florid complexion and dryness of the mouth. Each corresponded to a certain excess, that of *yin* in the case of the cold syndrome and that of *yang* in the case of the hot syndrome. The former was treated with 'hot' drugs, thereby providing *yang* to drive out the cold, and the latter was treated with 'cold' drugs. The syndromes associated with depletion and excess were evidence of either a lack or surfeit of energy.

The three opposing principles of external-internal, cold-hot and depletion-excess were the morbid expression of antinomic phenomena identified with *yin* (internal, cold, depletion) or *yang* (external, hot, excess), all part of a dual system in which imbalance caused illness. Physicians referred to a *yin* or *yang* syndrome. The first was manifested by depletion and cold, the second by excess and heat.

Ming Wong notes that the symptoms revealed by these eight principles or syndromes 'allowed one to forestall illness'; moreover, 'they indicated the required treatment'.[4] A state of depletion, for example, required an invigorating treatment. Invigoration (*bu*) was one of the eight therapeutic methods of traditional Chinese medicine; besides sweating (*han*), vomiting (*tu*) and purging (*xia*) already referred to, there was resort to harmonisation (*he*), warming (*wen*), purification (*qing*) and dispersion (*xiao*), all of which had been practised since the time of Zhang Zhongjing and the *Shanghanlun*. Sweating, vomiting and purging were important for a physician like Zhang Congzheng, who, in order to eliminate external pathogenic factors (wind, cold, humidity, heat), relied as much on gymnastic exercises as on drugs to induce sweating.

According to traditionalists, all drugs were endowed with certain properties: cold (*han*), hot (*re*), warm (*wen*) or cool (*liang*), and sometimes neutral (*ping*). A particular drug could also be acid, bitter, acrid, salty and even insipid (*dan*). Each drug was linked (*gui*: 'to belong to') to a certain meridian (channel), which itself was connected with a particular organ. The *yin* meridians (*taiyin, shaoyin, jueyin*) corresponded to the lungs, spleen, heart, kidneys and liver, while the *yang* meridians (*yangming, taiyang, shaoyang*) corresponded to the large intestine, stomach, small intestine, bladder, 'triple burner' and gall-bladder. Thus the rhizome of the *Alpinia officinarum* was considered a drug with acrid and hot qualities that worked on the meridians connected with the spleen and stomach, and the root of the *Scutellaria baicalensis* was a drug with bitter and cold qualities that worked on the meridians connected with the lungs, liver, stomach and large intestine.

Liu Wansu, Founder of the Hejian School

Liu Wansu (1110/1120–1200) was a native of Hejian, a district in present-day Hebei province. Called Master Hejian, or simply Liu Hejian, he bequeathed his name to a school of which he was the founder. Although the Zhangzong emperor (1189–1208) of the Jin dynasty invited Liu Wansu on three occasions to take up an official post, he refused, preferring to practise medicine among the people. He in fact became one of the most talented physicians during the Jin dynasty. The authors of *A History of Chinese Medicine* consider that he 'stretched the limits of medicine during the Jin and Yuan periods',[5] and, indeed, he played a highly significant role in the history of Chinese medicine. He was the author of several works based on the *Suwen* (*Essential Questions of the Huangdi Neijing*), the most representative being the *Suwen Xuanji Yuanbingshi*, in which he outlined his pathogenic concepts, and the *Huangdi Suwen Xuanming Fanglun*, which is of special interest for its discussion of therapy. He also wrote the *Suwen Bingji Qiyi Baomingji* (Li Shizhen in the sixteenth century disputed Liu's authorship and attributed the work to Liu's colleague Zhang Yuansu) and the *Shanghan Zhige Lunfang*, which deals principally with cold-induced (*Shanghan*) illnesses.

The basis of Liu Wansu's aetiological and therapeutic approach was the so-called theory of the 'five movements' (*yun*) and 'six influences' (*qi*). The *Suwen*, to which Liu referred, maintained that the five elements (wood, fire, earth, metal, water) controlled all phenomena. It was changes among them, Ming Wong observes, 'that determined life or death, growth or decay, health or sickness'.[6] The term *yun* ('to turn') referred to the 'movements' carried out by these five elements. The 'six influences' referred to the wind (*feng*), heat (*re*), humidity (*shi*), fire (*huo*), drought (*zao*) and cold (*han*). They were in some way the manifestation of the environment from which an illness might ensue. Thus what one would describe today as a windy dyspepsia would have been attributed in Liu Wansu's day to the influence of humidity. In the preface to the *Suwen Xuanji Yuanbingshi*, Liu Wansu writes: 'The doctrine of change is based on the five elements and the eight trigrams, Confucian doctrine is based on the three rules and five virtues, and medical doctrine is based on the five movements and six influences'.[7]

Liu Wansu's novel contribution was to accord prominence to fire and heat among the six influences; according to Liu, most pathological change resulted from these two influences, and he therefore tended to recommend the use of drugs with cold or cool qualities.

Zhang Yuansu, Master of the Yishui School

Like his older contemporary, Liu Wansu, Zhang Yuansu also came from Hebei province. Like Liu also, the school which he founded was named after his native district, Yishui. His *Yixue Qiyuan* (*Explanation of Medicine*), published in 1186 for the benefit of his followers, embodied Zhang's thought and experience. He considered that 'the prescriptions of the past were not appropriate for the illnesses of today'.

Nevertheless, Zhang Yuansu did not reject the teachings of his predecessors, and he relied especially on the *Huangdi Neijing*, the *Nanjing*, the *Shanghanlun* and the *Zongzangjing* (mentioned previously in connection with Hua Tuo) to form his own medical concepts. For Zhang, illness was a manifestation of the functional imbalance of the *zang* and *fu* organs. It was thus from the pathological condition revealed by these organs that Zhang determined the cause and nature of an illness, thereby arriving at a diagnosis. An appropriate therapeutic method would then follow. Zhang Yuansu also promoted the idea that medical drugs had a specific effect on the meridians with which they were associated.

Li Gao and the *Treatise on the Spleen and Stomach*

Nicknamed 'the old gentleman of the Eastern Wall', Li Gao (1180–1251) came from a wealthy family. His biographers make a special point of emphasising that medicine and pharmacy fascinated him from childhood. In any event, Li Gao's master was Zhang Yuansu, then practising medicine at Yizhou (present-day Yishui). Li's medical writings include the *Neiwaishang Bianhuolun* (*Treatise on the Differentiation between Endogenous and Exogenous Diseases*), the *Piweilun* (*Treatise on the Spleen and Stomach*) and the *Lanshi Micang* (*Secret Treasure from the Chamber of Orchids*).

Li Gao's writings reveal a physician's preoccupation with the effects of lifestyle on the body's organs. For Li, immoderation and intemperance affected principally the spleen and stomach, which he considered to be the 'root' of the 'original influence' (*yuanqi*), that is the principle of life or vitality. If the spleen and stomach were 'injured' (the literal translation of *shang*, as in *shanghan*: 'cold that injures', 'an attack of cold'), vitality would wither; this weakening of the original influence would then cause illness. This theory was outlined in Li Gao's most important work, the *Piweilun*: 'If the *qi* of the spleen and stomach is affected, then the original *qi* cannot carry out its function; this is the cause of illness'. Li Gao's psychosomatic approach to illness (he maintained that joy, anger, sadness, grief, fear and apprehension could all adversely affect the original *qi*), reflected a society overwhelmed by the effects of war, oppression, famine, poverty (in Chinese translated as 'crushed by hunger and cold') and epidemics.

Since the weakening of the original *qi*, in Li Gao's view, was the origin of illness, it is not surprising that Li especially recommended the use of tonics, the most important of which was ginseng. Others that were often prescribed included the root of the *Astragalus membranaceus*, the rhizome of *Glycyrrhiza uralensis*, the root of the *Angelica sinensis* and that of the *Ophiopogon japonicus*.

The Followers of the Yishui School

The teachings of the Yishui School were carried on by Wang Haogu and Luo Tianyi. Wang Haogu, born around 1200, studied under Zhang and then Li Gao. Their influence on Wang's medical thought was evident in his *Yinzheng Lueli*, a work devoted to what has been described above as the *yin* syndrome (*yinzheng*). Wang Haogu also wrote the *Yilei Yuanrong*, the *Tangye Bencao*, one of the materia medica of the Yuan period, and the *Cishi Nanzhi*, an account of the teachings acquired from his master, Li Gao.

The reasons for Wang's particular emphasis on the *yin* syndrome are to be found in the *Yinzheng Lueli*: 'The *yang* syndrome is easy to distinguish and therefore not difficult to treat; the *yin* syndrome is less easy to distinguish and therefore is difficult to treat'. Wang

Haogu therefore concentrated on achieving a better understanding
of the symptoms associated with the *yin* syndrome and on devising
an appropriate therapy to treat the illnesses identified with the three
yin meridians (*taiyin, shaoyin, jueyin*).

Luo Tianyi was another of Li Gao's disciples who achieved
renown during the eighth century. In his *Weisheng Baojian* (*Precious
Mirror of Health*), he supplemented Li Gao's medical theories with
his own observations.

Zhang Congzheng and the Theory of the 'Six Doors' and 'Three Methods'

Like Zhang Yuansu, Zhang Congzheng (c. 1150–1228) considered
that 'the prescriptions of former times could not completely cure the
illnesses of today'. Such a statement testified to the reforming spirit
of this military physician who, on his return home, compiled a work
(with the collaboration of Ma Zhiji and Chang Zhongming) based
on his observations and research, entitled the *Rumen Shiqin*. As the
title suggested, it was written for the benefit of scholars (*rumen*).

Zhang is known for his theory of the 'six doors' (*men*) and 'three
methods' (*fa*). The six doors referred to the six influences first
described by Liu Wansu. The three methods referred to sweating,
vomiting and purging, which meant, as far as therapy was
concerned, crucial importance being attached to the use of sudorifics,
emetics and purgatives, all of which Zhang prescribed in a large
number of cases. He maintained that, in order to treat an illness, the
evil (*xie*) influences had to be expelled; the *Huangdi Neijing*, in fact,
had already referred to such evil influences: 'They attack the centre
and its orifices'.[8] These evil influences were pathogenic agents that
Zhang Congzheng grouped into three distinct categories: 'harmful
influences of heaven' (wind, cold, heat, dampness, dryness and
fire), 'harmful influences of the earth' (fog, dew, rain, hail, ice and
mud) and 'harmful influences of man' (i.e. in food and drink: sour,
bitter, mild, acrid, salty and insipid). Zhang saw himself in the
forefront of an attack (*gong*) against these influences, convinced
that, once they had been eliminated, 'good health will be restored of
itself'.

To achieve this, Zhang gave preference to the three methods
mentioned above (and recommended earlier by the *Shanghanlun*).
He recommended sweating to eliminate the harmful influences
affecting the body's surface: 'The influences of wind, cold, dampness
and heat penetrate the skin but not deeply. To expel them quickly
there is nothing better than to make the patient sweat.' According to
Zhang, several methods could achieve this result, for example the

resort to fumigation or *daoyin* gymnastic exercises, but what is of special interest is Zhang's use of drugs administered in the form of decoctions (*Cinnamomum cassia, Ephedra sinica, Pueraria lobata, Cimicifuga foetida, Bupleurum chinense*) or powder. He listed a total of forty sudorific drugs, certain of which (besides those just mentioned) are still used today, such as *Schizonepeta tenuifolia* and *Angelica dahurica*.[9]

The second of Zhang's methods was induced vomiting. Included among the emetics he recommended were the root of the *Dichroa febrifuga* and the flower-stalk of the *Cucumis melo*, which Zhang Zhongjing had earlier prescribed in the form of powder.[10] When it came to the method of purging, Zhang Congzheng had a choice of thirty plants with purgative qualities, among which was the rhubarb, appreciated by Chinese therapists from antiquity to the present.[11] He also used the kernel of the *Prunus japonica*, the root of the *Euphorbia kansui* and the seeds of *Croton tiglium*. In the *Rumen Shiqin*, Zhang also gave warning advice: no purging, for example, in the case of recurrent dysentery. Moreover, he had a certain mistrust of invigoration, although he did not rule it out completely.

Zhu Zhenheng and his Minister of Fire

A native of Yiwu in Zhejiang province, Zhu Zhenheng (1281–1358) is also known as Master Danxi ('River of Cinnabar'). Such a sobriquet might indicate that he practised alchemy, but in fact it referred to the river beside which he lived. After studying under a scholastic master of the time, a follower of Zhu Xi's philosophy, Zhu Zhenheng discovered medicine on reading the *Suwen*. He then undertook a systematic study of the field.

The *Gezhi Yulun* was the fruit of his 'in-depth research' (the translation of *gezhi*), the essential points of which can be summarised as follows: *yang* is synonymous with movement and therefore change; *yin* is synonymous with rest, and therefore harmony. From this interaction come water, fire, wood, metal and earth. Fire has two phases, known as 'master-fire' (*jun*) and 'minister-fire' (*xiang*). Fire 'presides over everything that is in movement, therefore everything that is in movement comes from fire'. The 'fire' of the body is revealed during the course of physiological or pathological change. The 'minister-fire' refers to the energy that drives the body and is principally present in the liver and kidneys. Its immoderate action is harmful since it consumes *yin*: 'when *yin* weakens, illness arises; when *yin* is exhausted, death ensues'. Moreover, Zhu Zhenheng notes, when *yang* is in 'surplus', *yin* becomes 'insufficient'. This is one of the essential points of

Zhu's doctrine. To simplify, one can speak of the 'minister-fire' syndrome caused by the loss of *yin* energy associated with the liver and kidneys. The appropriate therapy thus had to make up for this deficiency by 'nurturing *yin*'. Such an idea appears in other works by Zhu Zhenheng such as the *Danxi Xinfa*, the *Jingui Guoxuan* and the *Jufang Fahui* (*fahui*: 'to explain one's ideas and feelings'), in which he discussed the problems arising in his view from the well-known book on prescriptions compiled during the Song (the *Taiping Huimin Heji Jufang*). He also wrote the *Bencao Buyi* (*Supplementary Materia Medica*).

Acupuncture, Treatment of Furunculosis and Abscesses, and the Setting of Fractures

The name of Dou Hanqing (Dou Jie), born around 1232, is familiar to Chinese acupuncturists. His tract, entitled the *Zhenjing Zhinan* is one of the *Four Books of Acupuncture and Moxibustion* (*Zhenjiu Sishu*) published in 1331 by Dou Guifang. The other three are the *Huangdi Mingdang Jiujing*, a treatise on moxibustion whose author is unknown but which was written before the Song period; the *Jiu Gaohuang Shuxuefa*, a manual on the application of moxas to the *gaohuang* (region of the body between the heart and diaphragm) by Zhuang Chuo, who lived during the Song; and the *Ziwuliuzhu Zhenjing* by He Ruoyu, an acupuncturist during the Jin dynasty.[12]

The *Huangdi Mingdang Jiujing* is a general description of moxibustion that outlines the various points (or locations) on the body to which it can be applied, and their corresponding therapeutic virtues. The point known as *yongquan* ('gushing spring'), for example, is situated at the lower end of the arch of the foot and its therapeutic virtue, according to the *Huangdi Mingdang Jiujing*, lies in the treatment of 'praecordial pain, loss of appetite, female sterility, coughing, shortness of breath, pharyngitis . . . headaches and blackouts . . .'.[13]

Another example given concerns the point known as *jiuwei* ('tail of the turtle-dove'), used in the treatment of 'palpitations . . . and epilepsy'. A contemporary handbook on acupuncture and moxibustion, *A Summary of Chinese Acupuncture*, confirms this since it indicates the same point for the treatment of 'heartburn, gastralgia, vomiting, hiccups, epilepsy, psychosis'.[14]

Finally, with regard to children – the second part of *Huangdi Mingdang Jiujing* is devoted to the use of moxibustion on children – the point known as *zhongting* ('grand hall of the centre') deserves mention. An acupuncturist today makes use of this point to treat infant regurgitation.[15] The *Huangdi Mingdang Jiujing* has similar

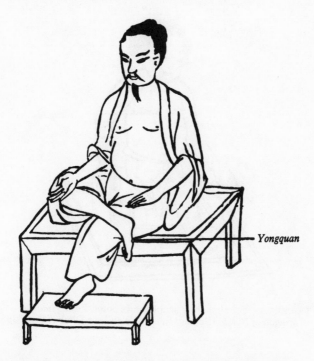

FIGURE 7.1   The *yongquan* acupuncture point. From *Huangdi Mingdang Jiujing* (Beijing: Renmin Weisheng Chubanshe, 1983).

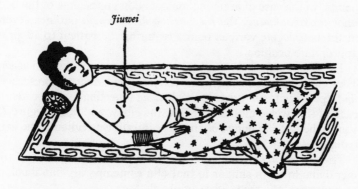

FIGURE 7.2   The *jiuwei* acupuncture point. From *Huangdi Mingdang Jiujing* (Beijing: Renmin Weisheng Chubanshe, 1983).

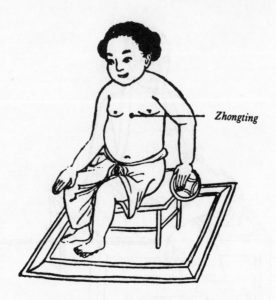

FIGURE 7.3   The *zhongting* acupuncture point. From *Huangdi
Mingdang Jiujing* (Beijing: Renmin Weisheng Chubanshe, 1983).

advice: 'If the child throws up its milk, apply moxibustion to the
zhongting point at the rate of one *zhuang* (i.e. one unit of ignited
artemesia)'.

Various procedures exist to locate acupuncture and moxibustion
points. In the case of applying moxibustion on the area of the body
known as *gaohuang*, the *Jiu Gaohuang Shuxuefa* outlines several
methods to locate various points requiring the patient to adopt an
appropriate position.

The *Ziwuliuzhu Zhenjing* discusses the five points known as *shu*.
These special points, which are called *jing* ('pit'), *rong* ('efflorescence'),
jing ('passage'), *shu* ('transport') and *he* ('meeting'), are located on
each of the twelve meridians below the elbow and knee. Figure 7.4
shows the five *shu* points on the large intestine meridian of the hand
(*yangming*).

The *Ziwuliuzhu Zhenjing* also describes the course of the
meridians in ways similar to that of a contemporary handbook on
acupuncture. We read, for example, that

    the large intestine meridian of the hand starts from the end of
    the index-finger, proceeds along the finger, passes between two
    bones at the point known as *hegu*, crosses two tendons, then

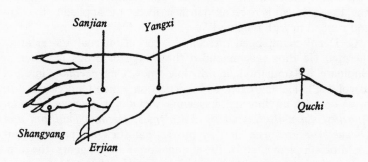

FIGURE 7.4   The *shu* points on the large intestine meridian of the hand (*yangming*). From *Ziwuliuzhu Zhenjing* (Beijing: Renmin Weisheng Chubanshe, 1983).

proceeds along the arm to the external side of the elbow, up the arm to the shoulder ... then descends to the cavity of the upper collar-bone (*quepen*), meets up with the lungs, crosses the diaphragm and finally links up with the large intestine.[16] Among the disorders associated with this meridian, the *Ziwuliuzhu Zhenjing*, like the *Summary of Chinese Acupuncture* today, points to toothache, nosebleeds and pharyngitis.

The most important name in the field of external medicine during the Yuan is most certainly that of Qi Dezhi (fourteenth century), whose *Waike Jingyi* (*The Essentials of External Medicine*) dates from 1335. He believed that the presence of abscesses, boils and, in general, all kinds of purulent inflammation had a close connection with the body as a whole. They arise, he wrote, 'from the imbalance of *yin* and *yang*'.[17] The first half of Qi's work outlines various therapeutic methods involving minor surgery, while the second half draws up a list of remedies making use of decoctions, pills, powders and ointment.

The *Waike Jingyi* is more a work on dermatology than on surgery per se. Its chief interest lies in the 145 remedies to treat all kinds of cutaneous illnesses. Dry and flaky skin, for example, is treated by an ointment known as 'ointment of heavenly hemp'. One of its ingredients is precisely *tianma* ('heavenly hemp'), the vernacular name for *Gastrodia elata*.[18] Other ingredients of this ointment are *Aconitum carmichaeli, Veratrum nigrum* and *Ligusticum wallichii*. As with the other remedies outlined in the *Waike Jingyi*, details are given of its preparation: the ingredients are to be fried in a little oil, left to cool, strained, blended with beeswax and pork grease, strained again, and then calomel (*qingfen*: 'light powder') added. Finally, how the ointment is to be used is described: 'it is applied to the skin and rubbed in with the hand'.

Qi Dezhi championed the combination of internal and external therapy. He thus recommended the intake of drugs in order to eliminate inflammation, a principle known as *neixiao* ('internal dissolving'). The ingredients of a decoction which Qi prescribed to bring on such an 'internal dissolving' included *Cimicifuga foetida*, *Angelica sinensis*, *Scutellaria baicalensis*, *Paeonia lactiflora* and *Glycyrrhiza uralensis*. If this proved insufficient, the treatment could be supplemented by the elimination of toxic agents (the term used is *du*: 'poison') with the aid of drugs to fortify vital energy and the blood, such as the 'powder of internal support' (*neituo san*) prescribed for a weakened condition. Besides *Angelica sinensis* and *Ligusticum wallichii*, this powder contained *Platycodon grandiflorum*, *Ledebouriella divaricata* and, of course, *Panax ginseng*. Phytotherapy was an integral component of Qi Dezhi's therapy. His 'decoction to dissolve poison' contained nearly forty medicinal plants, as did his 'ointment of ten perfumes' prescribed for the treatment of boils, anthrax, scrofulous tumours, haemorrhoids and even subcutaneous nodules.

Qi Dezhi's contemporary, Wei Yilin (c. 1277–1347), was more interested in orthopaedics. Skilled in setting fractures and in treating dislocations of the shoulder, hips and knee, Wei Yilin on occasion made use of anaesthetic drugs. His book *Shiyi Dexiaofang* (*Efficacious Remedies of the Physicians*) testifies not only to his proficiency in the field of orthopaedics but also in laryngology, stomatology, odontology, ophthalmology, gynaecology and obstetrics.

Wise Ways of Eating and Drinking

It is to a Mongol, Hu Sihui, that China owes the *Yinshan Zhengyao* (*Important Principles of Food and Drink*), published in 1330. As a dietician, Hu Sihui championed the idea that good health arose from a balanced diet. The people of antiquity, he wrote at the outset, 'took as their guide to life the harmony between *yin* and *yang* . . . they observed moderation in eating and drinking'. Yet the people of today, he continued, 'are ignorant of what to avoid in their diet, and they pay no heed to moderation'. Pointing out that by the time they reached fifty, people were afflicted with numerous maladies, Hu Sihui reiterated the basic rule of 'neither too much nor too little', a rule which he applied to sexual activity as much as to eating and drinking.

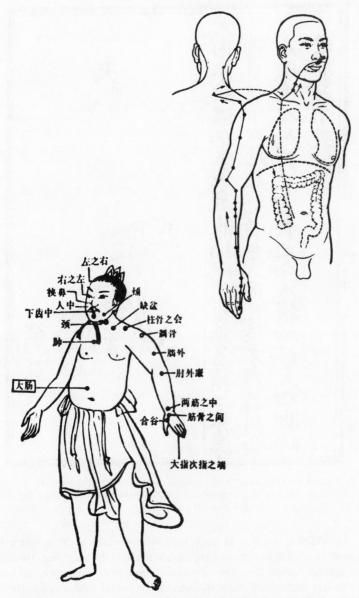

FIGURE 7.5   The large intestine meridian of the hand (*yangming*).
Above, from *Summary of Chinese Acupuncture* (Beijing: Waiwen
Chubanshe, 1977). Below, from *Ziwuliuzhu Zhenjing* (Beijing:
Renmin Weisheng Chubanshe, 1983).

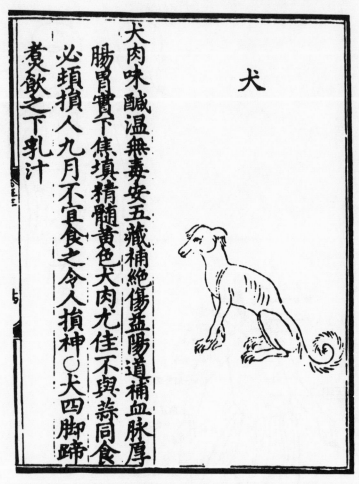

FIGURE 7.6   Dogmeat, 'salty, not too overpowering, and non-toxic, calms the five *zang* organs . . .'. From *Yinshan Zhengyao* (Beijing: Beijingshi Zhongguo Shudian, 1985).

In addition to offering such recommendations as 'it is better to brush the teeth in the evening rather than in the morning, thereby avoiding toothache', the *Yinshan Zhengyao* suggests various remedies and, most notably, provides a list of 230 cereals, meat, fish, shellfish, fruits and vegetables with a description of their dietary benefits. The book also gives advice on healthy eating. Thus the apple (*naizi, Malus asiatica*) is 'bitter and cold. If one eats too many the stomach will be distended. A sick person should not eat any.' Dogmeat, which is 'salty, not too overpowering, and non-toxic, calms the five *zang* organs', while deermeat 'fortifies the five *zang* organs' and 'boosts energy'. Grapes also sustain energy; moreover, they 'strengthen character'. A warning is raised against eating too many oranges, since they 'bring harm to the liver'. Likewise, too many bamboo shoots will cause illness.[19]

How to Cure Tuberculosis, Treat Sick Children and Nourish the Vital Principle

The name of Ge Kejiu, or Ge Qiansun (1305–52), is associated with the treatment of pulmonary tuberculosis, about which he wrote an entire work, the *Shiyao Shenshu*, in 1348. The book contains the remedies to cure the disease, or at least to slow down its progression, with the aid of powders, decoctions and pills (administered in a certain order). The field of paediatrics, which had begun to flourish during the Song dynasty, was represented in the Mongol period by Zeng Shirong, whose *Houyou Xinshu* dates from 1294. Besides a section on theory and clinical observation, the book contains 230 prescriptions. Finally, mention must be made of Cheng Wuji, the Jin-dynasty expert on the *Shanghanlun* (referred to in the previous chapter), and Qiu Chuji (born in the thirteenth century), a Daoist monk who founded the celebrated White Cloud Temple near Beijing and who was preoccupied with devising remedies and exercises to 'nourish the vital principle'.

Notes

1. Jacques Gernet, *A History of Chinese Civilization*, op. cit., p 368.
2. On aconite, see the excellent study by N. G. Bisset, 'Arrow Poisons in China', *Journal of Ethnopharmacology*, 1979, 1981. Bisset shows that poison arrows were used in China at least 2,500 years ago, and that the principal ingredient of the poison was an extract from tubercles of the *Aconitum*, in particular *Aconitum carmichaeli*. For the period under discussion, Bisset notes with regard to the Mongols' attempted invasion of Japan: 'The invading forces comprised Mongols, Chinese and Koreans, and, according to Japanese testimony, various types of poisoned arrows were included in the weapons used' (p 336).
3. Maurice-Robert Coyaud, *Les Opéras des Bords de l'Eau – Théâtre Yuan* (Paris: Centre National de la Recherche Scientifique, 1975), vol. 1, p 40.
4. Ming Wong, *La Médecine Chinoise par les Plantes*, op. cit., p 65.
5. *Zhongguo Yixueshi*, op. cit., p 71.
6. Ming Wong, *La Médecine Chinoise par les Plantes*, op. cit., p 77.
7. *Suwen Xuanji Yuanbingshi* (Nanjing: Jiangsu Kexue Jishu Chubanshe, 1985), p 7. The 'doctrine of change' refers to the *Yijing* (*Classic of Changes*). The three rules govern the relationship between ruler and subject, father and son, husband

and wife. The five virtues refer to humanity, justice, decorum, wisdom and sincerity.

8. Translation by Claude Larre and Elisabeth Rochat de La Vallée, *Assaisonner les Esprits*, op. cit., p 3. In this interpretive essay on the *Huangdi Neijing Suwen*, the authors note that these evil influences invade 'all the hollows and cavities where life is concentrated and nourished'. The *Xiandai Hanyu Cidian* (*Dictionary of Contemporary Chinese*) (Beijing: Shangwu yin-shuguan, 1979), p 1262, defines the term *xie* as: 'In Chinese medicine it refers to the surrounding factors that cause illness'.

9. These plants are included in the list of *jiebiaoyao*, literally 'drugs that disperse on the surface' (because they disperse evil influences to the surface of the body), noted in the *Zhongyixue Jichu*, op. cit., pp 86–94.

10. Catherine Despeux, op. cit., pp 91–2. On their use today in traditional Chinese medicine, see *Zhongyixue Jichu*, op. cit., pp 189–99.

11. Rhubarb (*Rheum palmatum, Rheum tanguticum, Rheum officinale*) heads the list of purgative drugs (*xiexiayao*) in *Zhongyixue Jichu*, op. cit., pp 95–6. For more details, see *Zhongyaozhi* (*Monograph on Chinese Drugs*) (Beijing: Renmin Weisheng Chubanshe, 1959, 1982), 1:24–35.

12. *Zhenjiu Sishu* (Beijing: Renmin Weisheng Chubanshe, 1983).

13. *Summary of Chinese Acupuncture*, op. cit., p 156, lists the following phenomena associated with the *yongquan* point: 'Coma, shock, mania, hysteria, epilepsy, infant convulsions, incoercible vomiting, pain in the crown of the head, pain in the throat, and dysuria'.

14. *Summary of Chinese Acupuncture*, op. cit., p 204.

15. Ibid.

16. Compare this description with the *Summary of Chinese Acupuncture*, op. cit., p 38.

17. *Waike Jingyi* (Nanjing: Jiangsu Kexue Jishu Chubanshe, 1985) p 1.

18. This plant, which belongs to the orchid family, grows at the expense of a mushroom, the *Armillaria mellea*. The *Gastrodia elata* (*tianma*) is referred to in the *Shen'nong Bancaojing* by the name of *chijian* ('red arrow'). It is mentioned again during the Song in the *Kaibao Bencao* (*Materia Medica of the Kaibao Era*), and then during the Ming in Li Shizhen's *Bencao Gangmu*. Pharmacological study of the *Gastrodia elata* has demonstrated its sedative and anticonvulsive properties, and it is used today in the treatment of vertigo, headaches and rheumatic pain. See Deng Shixan and Mo Yunjiang, *Acta Botanica Yunnanica*, 1 (2), 1979, pp 66–73.

19. *Yinshan Zhengyao* (Beijing: Beijingshi Zhongguo Shudian, 1985).

8

The Ming,
1368–1644

National Restoration

The two dates of 1368 and 1949 have an equal significance in the history of the Middle Kingdom. Not far from the Forbidden City constructed during the Ming between 1406 and 1429, Mao Zedong in 1949 solemnly proclaimed that 'The Chinese people have stood up'. The same words might well have been spoken by the founder of the Ming, Zhu Yuanzhang (reign name: Hongwu) after his victory over the Mongols. Moreover, as suggested by Jacques Gernet, one could compare the rehabilitation of the agrarian economy during Ming Hongwu's reign with that undertaken by the People's Republic after 1949. 'The priority accorded to the agrarian economy at the beginning of the Ming period', observes Gernet, 'seems to have been both a necessity and a deliberate choice. In a devastated China the most urgent thing was to ensure a food supply for the population. But at the same time a new direction was taken for the future: the Ming and Qing empires were to be mainly based on agriculture.'[1]

The political and economic restoration undertaken after 1368 was marred by an increasing trend towards autocracy. The dynasty's secret police was soon under the control of eunuchs, whose damaging influence continued to grow and was ultimately to lead to the dynasty's downfall. Nevertheless, the early Ming, in particular the reign of Yongle (1403–24), was a period of general prosperity. After seizing power by force from his nephew, the Jianwen emperor, Yongle ascended the throne and transferred the capital from Nanjing to Beijing. He then initiated the construction of the Forbidden City, the most impressive and best-preserved historical structure surviving in China today. This was also a time of the great maritime expeditions of Zheng He and the undertaking of encyclopaedic projects such as the *Yongle Dadian* (*Great Dictionary of the Yongle Reign*).

During the 1440s, the Mongols once again became a threat on China's northern frontiers. This threat intensified in the middle of the sixteenth century when Altan Khan laid siege to Beijing in 1550. At the same time, China's coasts were frequently prey to Japanese pirates (*wokou*). A century later, the Manchus became the new menace, imposing their rule over a weakened China beset by financial crisis, eunuch intrigues and popular insurrections such as the one led by Li Zicheng.[2] The end of the sixteenth century and the beginning of the seventeenth, however, witnessed an important reign, that of Wanli (1573–1619). It was during this period that the first cultural interaction between China and the West occurred.

The Jesuit Matteo Ricci (1552–1610) played a crucial role in this interaction. Arriving at the Portuguese enclave of Macao in 1582, he entered China the following year in the company of Michele Ruggieri. Yves Raguin notes that Ricci, who resided in Beijing from 1601 to 1610, brought with him 'cultural, as well as spiritual, knowledge',[3] translating, for example, Clavius's *Euclid's Geometry* into Chinese with the assistance of the scholar Xu Guangqi (1562–1633). Was this simply a ploy to attract interest in Christianity? In order to be accepted by the Chinese elite, Jacques Gernet writes, 'Ricci had to present himself as a moralist, philosopher and scholar'. However, Gernet continues, 'the strange thing that then came about was that, whereas the Jesuits had sought to use the prestige of the sciences in Europe to reinforce the authority of religion, the Chinese rejected that religion, wishing to retain only the scientific knowledge'.[4]

The word Ming conjures up in many minds an original and varied style of ceramics, but it should not be forgotten that the Ming period also saw the publication of important literary works such as *Jin Ping Mei* (*The Golden Lotus*) and *Xiyouji* (*Journey to the West*). The most renowned philosophers of the time were Wang Yangming (1472–1528), who influenced physicians like Zhang Jiebin, and Li Zhi (1527–1602), celebrated for his nonconformism. One of Wang Yangming's key sayings was: 'There is no principle (*li*) or object outside the mind', meaning that moral truth was to be found within oneself.

A Western View of Chinese Medicine

With their first-hand accounts of China, the Jesuits responded to the curiosity shown by Europeans in the seventeenth and eighteenth centuries concerning the nature of other cultures. What do their writings reveal about Chinese medicine? In the third chapter of the *Histoire de l'Expédition Chrétienne au Royaume de la Chine* (*A*

History of the Christian Expedition to the Kingdom of China),
Matteo Ricci and Nicolas Trigault refer to Chinese medical practice
in the sixteenth and seventeenth centuries:

> China is rich in medicinal herbs which are known elsewhere
> only as importations. Rhubarb and musk were first brought in
> from the West by the Saracens, and after spreading through
> the whole of Asia, they were exported to Europe at an almost
> unbelievable profit . . . Here, too, you find that famous remedy
> for many diseases, called Chinese Wood by the Portuguese and
> Sacred Wood by others. It grows freely in barren parts and
> without cultivation, and may be obtained for the price of the
> labour necessary to collect it, but it is exported at a high price.[5]

Elsewhere, Ricci and Trigault acknowledged that

> the art of medicine in China differs very much from what we
> are accustomed to. Their method of taking the pulse, however,
> is the same as ours and they are quite successful in bringing
> about cures. In general, they make use of very simple remedies
> such as herbs and roots and other such things. In fact, the
> whole art of Chinese medicine is practically contained in the
> rules we ourselves follow for the use of herbs.[6]

On the other hand, Ricci and Trigault observe with astonishment
that 'no-one is prohibited from attempting to cure the sick, whether
he be skilled in medicine or not'.[7]

Finally, if they condemn without reservation 'the stupidity of
alchemy' and 'the sellers of immortality', Ricci and Trigault are less
judgmental when discussing the cure of sickness through baptism.[8]

A Medical Encyclopaedia

The *Yongle Dadian* (*Great Dictionary of the Yongle Reign*),
completed in 1408, originally comprised 22,877 entries. Only 795
survive today, of which seventy-two are of particular interest for
medicine and pharmacy.[9] These provide a clear idea of the interest
taken in this domain. Thus the section on 'children's nosebleeds'
contains first of all a list of bibliographical references, citing the
Zhubing Yuanhoulun (*Treatise on the Causes and Symptoms of
Illness*) by Chao Yuanfang, the *Qianjin Yaofang* (*Prescriptions of
the Thousand Ounces of Gold*) by Sun Simiao, and the *Shengji
Zonglu* (*General Catalogue of Divine Assistance*). This is then
followed by a description of a number of remedies culled from
various sources such as the *Taiping Shenghuifang*. The section
devoted to the plum is crammed with extracts from various materia
medica such as the *Shen'nong Bencaojing* and Su Song's *Tujing*

Bencao (*Illustrated Materia Medica*). The *Yongle Dadian* also brings together medical texts such as the *Shanghanlun*, which is richly annotated with commentaries by, for example, the Song expert Cheng Wuji.

The Treasure of the 'River of Cinnabar'

The treasure of the 'river of cinnabar' refers to the legacy bequeathed by Zhu Zhenheng (d. 1358), alias Danxi ('river of cinnabar'), to two of his disciples, Wang Lu and Dai Sigong. Wang and Dai completed Zhu's theoretical work on the consequences arising from the weakening of *yin*.

A native of Kunshan in Jiangsu province, Wang Lu (c. 1332–91) belonged to the group of physicians who, in the wake of Liu Wansu, Zhang Yuansu and others, believed that 'the prescriptions of former times could not cure the diseases of today'. An example of one such disease was the plague, which was introduced to China during the second century and attained epidemic proportions from the Song and Yuan periods onwards. Pang Anshi, who lived during the Song, reported that in 1090 'between spring and autumn people living in the two *jun* (an administrative division of the time) of Qi and Huang suddenly contracted sore throats' (*houbi*: 'obstruction of the throat'), and that death followed 'within twelve or twenty-four hours'. (There are other descriptions of this disease to which we shall return.) During the fourteenth century, Chinese physicians lacked the means to deal with this plague, and it was no doubt such helplessness in the face of such a disease, as well as other incurable afflictions, that prompted Wang Lu to go 'against the tide of accepted opinion on medical texts' in order to rediscover their original meaning. The title of one of his works, in fact, is the *Yijing Suhuiji* (*suhui*: 'to go against the tide'), which dates from 1368.

Thus Wang Lu sought to retrace the original lessons of the *Shanghanlun* after noting the confusion that then existed between *shanghan* (cold-induced illness) and *wenbing* (febrile illness). Those who diagnosed *wenbing* as if it were *shanghan*, he wrote, did not respect Zhang Zhongjing's original intention. What did the author of *Shanghanlun* have to say on this? 'When, in the case of an illness associated with the *taiyang* meridian, a patient is feverish, thirsty, and is not susceptible to cold, one can speak of a "febrile" illness.'[10] In order to understand Wang Lu's novel approach, a brief historical summary of the notion of *wenbing* is in order. Wang Shuhe, promoter of Chinese pulsing during the third century, distinguished five kinds of *shanghan*, later to be increased to nine. From the time the *Huangdi Neijing* appeared to the Northern Song, it would seem that *shanghan* was the generic term used to describe all types of febrile illness, *wenbing* simply being one of the five or nine kinds of *shanghan*.[11]

With Pang Anshi, whose *Shanghan Zongbinglun* (*General Treatise on Shanghan*) was written around 1100, four kinds of *shanghan* were referred to as *wenbing*; such a change in vocabulary was meant merely to emphasise the evolution and gravity (even incurability) of the illness. It was only at the beginning of the Ming that the precise features and definition of *wenbing* were formulated. Wang Lu, who took the lead in this endeavour, recommended therapeutic cures for *wenbing* very different from those aimed at treating cases of *shanghan*.

Dai Sigong (1323-1405) is the author of a text with abundant references to the precepts of Zhu Zhenheng, of whom Dai was at once the faithful follower and creative successor. The title of Dai's work is revealing: *Tuiqiu Shiyi* (*A Thorough Examination of the Master's Medical Thought*). With its description of aetiology, symptomatology and therapeutic measures to treat fifty illnesses (or types of illness), the work is a valuable document for the study of the medical thought and practice of the Danxi school. The first of the three sections of the *Tuiqiu Shiyi*, entitled 'Various Illnesses', gives us an idea of the afflictions suffered by the Chinese during the fourteenth century: malaria, diabetes (the Chinese term *xiaoke* refers to the abnormal elimination of urine and intense thirst that characterise this condition), sore throat, cough, urticaria, tuberculosis, haemoptysis (spitting of blood), palsy, gonorrhoea, dysuria, diarrhoea, dysphagia (difficulty of swallowing) and arthralgia.

Among the clinical cases described in Dai's work is that of a woman suffering from appendicitis, diagnosed by a painful hardening on the right side of the navel and leading to a 'fever with cold shivers'. Moreover, 'the pain cannot be soothed since the pulse is full'. The patient 'will be cured in less than ten days' by draining the pus for three days with the use of a needle. Another interesting example concerns ejaculation of semen during sleep. The *Tuiqiu Shiyi* describes the case of a twenty-year-old insomniac who read every night until the small hours:

> Blood thereby does not return to the liver and as a consequence water in the kidneys is insufficient; fire therefore benefits from the lack of *yin* and enters into the lower burner, stimulating the sperm chamber. With containment of sperm no longer being possible, it escapes.

Various treatments are prescribed that will put an end 'within three months' to the involuntary emissions of sperm.[12]

The *Tuiqiu Shiyi* is also concerned with infant maladies such as ascarides (threadworm) (*huichong, Ascaris lumbricoides*), to be treated with 'drugs that kill worms', and the disease known as *gan*, whose symptoms reveal either a poor diet or parasites in the body. A third section of the work deals with gynaecology and obstetrics. It contains, for example, an account of the foetus: 'During the first month, the shape is formed; in the second month the substance; and in the third month sperm and blood are transformed into a foetus and the sex is differentiated'. A method to determine the sex of the foetus is also described:

> When a pregnant woman is in her dressing-room and someone calls to her suddenly from behind, if she turns her head to the left, she has a boy, if she turns her head to the right she has a girl. This is because a male is conceived in the left uterus and a female in the right uterus.

The School of Warming and Invigoration

If, as we have seen, Liu Wansu (founder of the Hejian school) and Zhu Zhenheng had their supporters during the Ming, they also aroused the opposition of physicians who adhered to the 'school of warming and invigoration' (*wenbu*).

The forerunner of this school was Xue Ji (c. 1488–1558). The son of a physician who had been a member of the official Academy of Medicine, Xue Ji began his medical career as a specialist in skin diseases (*yangyi*) before acquiring a reputation as a physician able to deal with all kinds of illness that required expertise in internal medicine, surgery, gynaecology, paediatrics and otorhinolaryngology. Xue Ji's writings are ample testimony to his wide medical interests. The *Neike Zhaiyao* (*A Summary of Internal Medicine*) is a companion piece to the *Waike Shuyao* (*Essentials of External Medicine*), itself completed by the *Waike Fahui* (*The Development of External Medicine*). Xue Ji was also the author of the *Nuke Cuoyao* (*A Résumé of Gynaecology*), the *Zhengti Leiyao* (*A Repertory of Traumatology*) and the *Kouchi Leiyao* (*A Repertory of Stomatology*), the earliest surviving Chinese treatise devoted exclusively to mouth and teeth complaints.

Xue Ji's therapy was based essentially on the principle of invigorating the spleen and kidneys with remedies such as the decoction borrowed from the *Jishengfang* (*Prescriptions to Save Life*) compiled by Yan Yonghe during the thirteenth century. Besides *panax ginseng*, the decoction comprised *Atractylodes macrocephela, Porio cocos, Astragalus membranaceus, Euphoria longana, Glycyrrhiza uralensis, Polygala tenuifolia, Angelica sinensis, Aucklandia lappa* and *Zizyphus spinosa*. Most of these herbal drugs 'belonged' (*gui*) to, or acted upon, the spleen meridian, hence the name of the decoction, *gui pi tang* ('decoction of drugs belonging to the spleen'). Xue Ji recommended it in his *Neike Zhaiyao* to treat amnesia, irregular periods and malaria.[13] He in fact devoted a whole chapter of the work to malaria. A few citations from the work show how such a disease was treated at the time: 'A scholar, having contracted a shivering fever during the autumn, had still not been cured by the spring'. Xue Ji made the patient take two ounces of ginseng and fresh ginger in order to bring the fever down. He then prescribed a 'decoction to regularise the middle burner and increase energy', comprising *Astragalus membranaceus, Panax ginseng, Glycyrrhiza uralensis, Atractylodes lancea, Bupleurum chinense, Cimicifuga foetida* and *Aucklandia lappa*, to which he added, in this case, *Pinellia ternata, Poria cocos* and *Zingiber officinale*. This same prescription, according to the *Neike Zhaiyao* (*A Summary of the* Huangdi Neijing), was given to a woman who, 'long afflicted with a shiverish fever', had lost her appetite. Xue Ji also recommended the decoction to treat inappetence and fatigue, at times prescribing instead a remedy known as the 'decoction to invigorate the middle burner and increase energy',[14] such as in the case of the malaria victim afflicted with fever, loss of appetite and fatigue. A single dose of this medicine would combat the fever, although complete recovery required several dosages.

Xue Ji recommended this decoction in many other cases:

A scholar one afternoon felt an irritation in the eyes, making it difficult to raise them. His health went into decline. I used the decoction to invigorate the middle burner and increase energy, supplementing it with ginseng and astragalus (milk-vetch). After taking it several times, the patient recovered completely.[15]

Xue Ji's herbal 'armoury' comprised older prescriptions such as the 'small decoction of hare's-ear' (a species of bupleurum) favoured by Zhang Zhongjing, and prescribed in the case of a man who 'felt pain in his penis' and who complained of urinary problems accompanied sometimes by itching.[16]

Historians of Chinese medicine usually consider Zhao Xianke as the supreme master of the *wenbu* ('to warm up, invigorate') school, of which Xue Ji was the founder. Zhao, born in the second half of the sixteenth century, expanded on the teachings of Xue Ji to formulate the theory of the 'gate of vitality' (*mingmen*: the area between the kidneys). According to Zhao, it was not the heart that governed the body but the 'gate of vitality', whose intensity or weakness of 'fire' corresponded with the expansion or diminution of energy. Insisting on the dual relationship between water, identified with *yin*, and fire, identified with *yang*, Zhao maintained that the physician had only to 'nourish' fire or water.

Zhao Xianke's teachings are outlined in the *Yiguan*. He treated his patients mainly with two kinds of pills known as 'the pill of eight ingredients', a prescription borrowed from Zhang Zhongjing's *Jingui Yaolue (Summary from the Golden Chest)* and 'the pill of six ingredients'; the former was prescribed to reinvigorate fire, while the latter was meant to reinvigorate water.[17]

If for Wang Yangming 'principle (*li*) is to be found in the mind', for Zhang Jiebin (also known as Zhang Jingyue: 1563–1640), whose medical theories were very much influenced by Wang's thought, '*yang* is life'. We have seen that Zhu Zhenheng had earlier maintained that *yang* as a rule was 'excessive' while *yin* was 'insufficient'. Zhang Jiebin denied that *yang* was excessive. It was, he claimed, the root of our physical existence and therefore was the source of life: 'Heat is *yang*, while cold is *yin*; the mildness of spring and summer is *yang*, the coldness of autumn and winter is *yin*'. Zhang concluded that it was during spring that everything was born and in summer that everything grew. Heat, identified with *yang*, was at the origin of the growth of the 10,000 beings. In the *yin-yang* dichotomy, therefore, *yang* occupied the key position. 'The life of the 10,000 beings comes from *yang*, the death of the 10,000 beings also derives from *yang* . . . The arrival of *yang* is life, while its disappearance is death.' Another theory favoured by Zhang Jiebin is summed up in the phrase: 'True *yin* is insufficient'. He prescribed, like Zhao Xianke, a pill based on *Rehmannia glutinosa* to treat a deficiency of *yin* and one based on *Aconitum carmichaeli* and *Cinnamomum cassia* to counter a fall in *yang*.

Zhang wrote a commentary to the *Huangdi Neijing* in which he grouped the text under twelve headings (e.g. 'Treatment of health', '*yin* and *yang*' and 'meridians'). For this reason, the commentary was entitled *Leijing (The Classified* Huangdi Neijing), and was published for the first time in 1624. His aim was to 'reveal what is hidden' and to 'simplify what is difficult'. It was completed in the same year by the *Leijing Fuyi (Supplement to the* Leijing) and an illustrated version, the *Leijing Tuyi*. Zhang's medical thought can also be found in two other works: the *Jingyue Quanshu (The Complete Work of Zhang Jiebin)*, which notably contains a critique of the theories of Liu Wansu and Zhu Zhenheng, and the *Zhiyilu (Questions to Clear up Doubts)*.

One Pox can Conceal Another

During the Ming, brothels did a roaring business, the more so, emphasises Robert van Gulik, when one considers that 'during the preceding periods promiscuous intercourse with courtesans and prostitutes had not involved the risk of incurring a fatal venereal disease'. Besides, van Gulik adds,

> the chances of infection were diminished by the cleanliness which the Chinese observed in their sexual habits. We know from the Ming erotic novels that men and women used to wash their private parts both before and after the coitus, and lubricants used such as agar-agar jelly covered up small wounds and abrasions on the genitals and prevented infection.[18]

These hygienic efforts were thwarted, however, by syphilis epidemics that raged during the sixteenth and seventeenth centuries. One can read in the *Xuyishuo* that 'during the last years of the Hongzhi era (1505) the population was afflicted with a terrible skin disease which began among the people of Guangdong (in the Canton region). As the people of Wu (the Yangzi region) were not affected, they called it Guangchuang ("Canton ulcers") or, because of its appearance, *yangmeichuang*' (*yangmei* was the vernacular name for the *Myrica rubra* tree).

Syphilis is mentioned in several medical works of the time, but it particularly attracted the attention of two physicians, Wang Ji and Chen Sicheng. Wang Ji (1463–1539) proved to be a doughty champion in the combat against syphilis. In accordance with his view that there could be no external treatment without internal treatment, he combined the use of decoctions and ointments. Thus he could prescribe a 'decoction of the four rulers' (*Panax ginseng, Atractylodes macrocephela, Poria cocos* and *Glycyrrhiza uralensis*) to sustain vital energy, while recommending the application of 'an ointment from the golden and silver flower' (*Lonicera japonica*: Japanese honeysuckle) on the patient's ulcers. At times, he also resorted to cauterisation using ignited garlic (*Allium sativum*). The cure would be completed by a treatment of 'recovery' using, for example, a 'decoction of the eight precious ingredients', which comprised those used in the 'decoction of the four rulers' as well as *Rehmannia glutinosa, Paeonia lactiflora, Angelica sinensis* and *Ligusticum wallichii*. This remedy is still used today in traditional Chinese medicine as a tonic for energy and for the blood.

For his part, Chen Sicheng, who lived during the late sixteenth and early seventeenth century, devoted an entire work to the treatment of syphilis, the *Meichuang Milu* (*Secret Writings on Putrid Ulcers*). Published in 1632, it was the first of its kind in China. Chen suggestively referred to syphilitic ulcers as 'fornication ulcers' and prescribed the use of arsenic and mercury to cure them.

Another scourge, dating from much earlier, preoccupied physicians of the time: smallpox. Although referred to in chapter 6, it is worth remembering that according to Yu Maokun, author of the *Douke Jinjing Fujijie* (*Explanation of Smallpox*) in the early eighteenth century, anti-smallpox vaccinations date from the years 1567–72.

Acupuncture on the Way to Success

The most important work on acupuncture and moxibustion during the Ming is the *Zhenjiu Dacheng* (*The Great Success of Acupuncture and Moxibustion*) by Yang Jizhou (1522–1620). Published in 1601, it brought together all essential knowledge in the field acquired over previous centuries, while at the same time drawing on Yang Jizhou's long experience to suggest new ways of using acupuncture. In 1561, for example, he successfully treated a paralysis of the lower limb by puncturing the *Huantiao* point located on the *shaoyang* gall-bladder meridian of the foot.[19] The *Zhenjiu Dacheng* was regularly reprinted during the seventeenth, eighteenth and nineteenth centuries, testifying to the enormous prestige it enjoyed.

By way of contrast, the *Zhenfang Liuji* (*Six Compositions on Acupuncture*), written in 1618 by Wu Kun (b. 1551), the well-known commentator on the *Suwen*, seems not to have enjoyed a similar reputation. Among other works on acupuncture during the Ming are the *Zhenjiu Daquan* (*Summary of Acupuncture and Moxibustion*) in 1439 by Xu Feng, the *Zhenjiu Wendui* (*Questions and Responses on Acupuncture and Moxibustion*) in 1530 by the surgeon, Wang Ji, and, especially, the *Zhenjiu Juying* (*The Best of Acupuncture and Moxibustion*) in 1529 by Gao Wu, which, along with Yang Jizhou's work, constituted the two most significant texts on acupuncture during the Ming period. In 1537, Gao Wu published another work, the *Zhenjiu Jieyao* (*Essentials of Acupuncture and Moxibustion*), which drew on the *Huangdi Neijing* and the *Nanjing* (*Classic of Difficult Problems*). The *Nanjing* was the subject of another study entitled *Nanjing benyi* (*The Original Meaning of the* Nanjing), whose author, Hua Shou (1304–86) was renowned as an acupuncturist. In 1341, he wrote the *Shisijing Fahui* (*An Explanation of the Fourteen Meridians*). Finally, Li Shizhen, of whom more will be said later, wrote a text in 1572 on the eight extra meridians.

Surgery Without a Scalpel

Wang Ji, also known as Shishan (Stone Mountain), whose role in the fight against syphilis and whose interest in acupuncture have already been noted, was against the excessive use of knives or needles. Wang, a follower of the Danxi school – his *Shishan Yi'an* (*Medical Treatises of Stone Mountain*) revealed the influence of Zhu Zhenheng's theories on his medical practice – outlined his thinking on surgery in a work dating from 1531, the *Waike Lili*. In essence, he maintained that, since the body was one entity, the treatment of a malady that required external medicine had to take into account (*zhi*: 'know', 'understand') the 'interior'. This was because, Wang continued, 'to treat the external (*wai*) while neglecting the internal (*nei*) is tantamount to not appreciating the origin (*ben*) of the sickness while being content to cure simply the external and final (*mo*) manifestation of the sickness'. Thus, Wang concluded, surgical instruments should not be used excessively. On the other hand, one should not hesitate to operate if it was absolutely necessary.

Wang Ji's contemporary, Xue Ji, insisted in his *Zhengti Leiyao* (*Repertory on Traumatology*) – besides expounding on the setting of fractures, this work, published in 1529, describes sixty-five cases of wounds caused by a blow, fall, weapon or boiling water – on the necessity of invigorating energy and blood, as well as on prescribing the appropriate cure for a patient. We have already seen how Wang Ji dealt with syphilitic ulcers, accompanying external treatment with a decoction to sustain energy.

The notion that external and internal treatment had to be harmoniously combined was shared by a number of physicians and surgeons during the Ming. They included Chen Shigong (1555–1636), one of the most outstanding figures in surgery at this time. His *Waike Zhengzong*, published for the first time in 1617, outlined a way of stitching the gash resulting from a suicide attempt to cut the throat: 'If the person is still breathing and the body is not already cold, it is advisable to stitch the gash immediately with silk thread'. The book also contains a description of cancer of the lip, which is said to manifest itself initially by a tumour the size of a kidney-bean. Then, attaining the size of a cocoon, the swelling becomes hard and painful. At this point, Chen Shigong declared the illness incurable. He suggested several causes for such a serious affliction; in addition to psychological factors such as profound distress – today we would speak more of depression – Chen spoke of localised inflammation due to the eating of fried, spicy or burnt food. Chen likewise described cancer of the breast. The tumour, he noted, is initially as big as a kidney-bean although it may not be too painful or itchy during the first years of the illness. Thereafter it gets bigger, and becomes more tender and ulcerous. The concave side of the tumour, according to Chen, is shaped like a hollow while the convex side resembles lotus seeds. The patient experiences extreme fatigue. Chen concluded that the illness at this stage was incurable.

Wang Kentang, a contemporary of Chen Shigong, described a case of breast cancer affecting a man who succumbed to depression following repeated failures in the civil service examinations. His left nipple began to ooze a small amount of liquid; shortly afterwards tumours appeared around the nipple, then swelled and became ulcerous. Wang declared the illness incurable.[20]

Surgery during the Ming benefited from development in the fields of anaesthesia (or rather analgesia), aseptic treatment and haemostasia. Among the new anaesthetic drugs used were a plant of the ericaceous family, *Rhododendron molle*, and jasmin, *Jasminum sambac*, which is known by its other usage as a scent for tea. Li Shizhen tried out a solanaceous plant, the *datura*, for its euphoric and calming effects, and recommended its use as a narcotic (*mayao*: *ma*, 'to make languid; *yao*, 'drug') when carrying out minor operations such as the lancing of an abscess.

Victims of the Plague

The word 'plague' is rendered in Chinese as *shuyi*, literally 'epidemic disease caused by rats', but during the Ming people spoke of *wenyi* ('pestilence'), that is any kind of fatal epidemic disease. It is known that in 1641 a plague epidemic decimated the populations of Hebei, Shandong, Jiangsu and Zhejiang. It is therefore no coincidence that Wu Youxing (who was born in the 1580s and died during the 1660s) focused on this disease in a book published in 1642, the *Wenyilun (On Pestilence)*. He described the specific features of various kinds of pestilence with reference to the generic term *shanghan* (described in chapter 3), and proposed the theory of 'excessive influences' (*liqi*), pathogenic agents responsible for the spread of pestilence (among which was included the 'pestilence of pustules', the term used by Wu Youxing for bubonic plague) and which penetrated the body through the 'mouth and nose'.

Moreover, Wu Youxing concluded that each of these pestilences was associated with its own particular 'excessive influence'. He distinguished 'pestilence among cattle' from that affecting chickens or even ducks, observing that animals, birds and humans could all fall prey to pestilence at different times. Wu Youxing's aetiological thesis that the origin of disease was due to multiple influences overturned medical thought of the time, which was generally inclined to emphasise the pathogenic influence of fire.

With regard to the plague, it might be noted that it was precisely on Chinese territory (in Hong Kong) that Alexander Yersin in 1894 discovered the bacillus of bubonic plague.

The Return of Spring, or Regained Health

The richness of imagery that the Chinese language possesses gives a special meaning to the titles of many medical works. The *Wanbing Huichun* by Gong Tingxian (1522–1619) is an example. The title of the work, which dates from 1587, associates the 'return of spring' (*hui*, 'return'; *chun*, 'spring') with the idea of recovering health after suffering one of the '10,000 illnesses' (*wan*, '10,000'; *bing*, 'illness') against which Gong Tingxian fought. Judging from the reputation which Gong acquired during his lifetime, in China and abroad (especially Japan, where the *Wanbing Huichun* was distributed from the beginning of the seventeenth century), such a struggle would appear to have been successful.

During the Ming, there was no lack of eminent physicians; a brief description of the following examples will be limited to essential aspects of their thought or practice. Lou Quanshan (1332–1401), in his *Yixue Gangmu* (*Compendium of Medicine*), emphasised the role of *yin* and *yang*, as well as the theory of the five elements. Wan Quan (or Wan Mizhai, 1495–1585), on the other hand, the author of over ten medical works, upheld the thesis in the *Youke Fahui* (*Explanation of Infant Illnesses*) that among children the liver was often in a state of excess (*youyu*: 'to be in excess') while the spleen was in a state of scarcity (*bu zu*, 'not sufficient'); he therefore tended to prescribe drugs to regularise and invigorate the spleen and stomach. Infant illnesses also attracted the attention of Wang Kentang, referred to earlier in connection with breast cancer. Wang was the author of a series of six specialised works grouped under the title of *Zhengzhi Zhunsheng*. One of them is specifically devoted to paediatrics, the five others dealing with 'diverse ailments', *shanghan* afflictions, 'illnesses of the skin' (the term for this category, *yang*, covered cutaneous affections like boils as well as wounds and burns), and gynaecology.

Chinese medicine at this time continued to rely on the traditional classics, beginning with the *Huangdi Neijing*. Li Zhongzi (1588–1655), for example, published the *Neijing Zhiyao*, one of several explanatory manuals on the *Huangdi Neijing*. There was also continued interest in the *Shanghanlun*; the *Shanghanlun Tiaobian* by Fang Youzhi (born in the sixteenth century) appeared in 1592, preceded in the middle of the fifteenth century by Tao Hua's *Shanghan Liushu* (*Six Books on the* Shanghanlun). Xiong Zongli (c. 1415–87) was drawn to the *Nanjing* (*Classic of Difficult Problems*); under the pseudonym of Wutingzi, he wrote the *Wutingzi Sujie Bashiyi Nanjing* (*Explanation of the Book of Eighty-one Difficult Problems*). General medical treatises were also published, such as the *Yizhong Bidu* (*What is Necessary to Study from the Medical Tradition*) in 1637 by Li Zhongzi, an eminent Shanghai physician. The *Yixue Rumen* (*Rudiments of Medicine*) by Li Jianzhai in 1575 aimed to be more didactic; it was republished several times during the Ming and Qing dynasties. Other general works included the *Yixue Zhengchuan* by Yu Tuan (1435–1517), a work that was profoundly influenced by Zhu Zhenheng and his school; the *Hanshi Yitong* (*Medical Synthesis of Master Han*) by Han Mao in 1522; the *Gujin Yitong* (*Synthesis of Past and Present Medicine*) by Xu Chunfu, which dates from 1556; and the *Yixue Liuyao* (*Six Important Points of Medicine*) by Zhang Sanxi (born in the sixteenth century).

The authors of these works were not content simply to expound theories but also aimed at offering practical advice. A quarter of *Hanshi yitong*, for example, which in a contemporary edition does not exceed forty pages, comprises various remedies.[21] An ophthalmologist like Ni Weide (1303–77) not only investigated why and how eyesight problems appeared but also proposed therapeutic measures to correct them. Moreover, new demands for efficacious advice were made at this time, and physicians such as Shen Zhiwen (sixteenth century) readily likened medical remedies to weapons of war.

Li Shizhen and the *Bencao Gangmu* (*Compendium of Materia Medica*)

Li Shizhen was born in 1518 in Waxiaba near Qizhou, which is situated in the present-day district of Qichun, Hubei province. He came from a family of physicians, the vocation often passing from father to son. Li's father, Li Yanwen, is known more for his knowledge than his skill as a medical practitioner. Li Yanwen's influence on the young Shizhen, nevertheless, soon stimulated in him an interest in medicine and pharmacy; from childhood he became acquainted with these fields, at first by working in the family herbalist's shop and then by accompanying his father to the patient's bedside. However, Li Yanwen had other ideas for his son's future and prodded him to aim for an official career, a more attractive prospect than that of a people's physician. Shizhen's repeated failures in the civil service examinations – the last one in 1540 – finally got the better of his father's ambitions. Li Shizhen had no other choice but to follow in his father's footsteps.

It appears that, early on, Li Shizhen thought of devising a materia medica free of the errors of his predecessors, of whom he undertook a close and methodical reading with the help of the *Zhenglei Bencao* (*Classified Materia Medica*) of Tang Shenwei, one of the most important herbalists during the Song dynasty. Li began work on the *Bencao Gangmu* in 1552, but, due to the complexity of the task, it was not completed until 1578. Recommended to the imperial court, Li departed in 1558 for Beijing, where he was admitted to the *Taiyiyuan* (Academy of Medicine), which brought together all the prominent medical figures of the time. Or at least this is what Li believed; his disappointment was to be bitter. He worked there for a year, taking advantage of his situation to study the readily-accessible medical writings. Then, using illness as a pretext, he took leave of his colleagues in the capital without regret. After a stay in Wuchang, he returned to Qizhou in 1561. From 1565 onwards, he travelled often in search of information, traversing the provinces of Henan, Hubei, Jiangxi, Jiangsu and Anhui. Once the *Bencao Gangmu* was completed, Li Shizhen in 1579 went to Nanjing, at that time a well-known centre for publishing. The work was not published until 1596, three years after Li Shizhen's death.

Li Shizhen wrote at least seventeen medical works,[22] but the only ones still extant are the *Bencao Gangmu*, the *Binhu Maixue* (*Binhu's Study of the Pulse*), which dates from 1564, and the *Qijing Bamai Kao* (*An Examination of the Eight Extra Meridians*), composed in 1572. However, it is as a herbalist that Li Shizhen attracts our interest.

The pharmaceutical work known as the *Bencao Gangmu* can be summarised under four aims: expanding the content of the materia medica, revising the classification of drugs, correcting errors in the works of Li's predecessors, and establishing guidelines for the preparation as well as the usage of drugs.

Out of the 1,892 drugs that the *Bencao Gangmu* lists, 1,518 were already known to Chinese herbalists: 347 had been mentioned for the first time in the *Shen'nong Bencaojing*, 306 in the *Shen'nong Bencaojing Jizhu* (*Annotations to the* Shen'nong Bencaojing) of Tao Hongjing, 111 in the *Tang Bencao* of Su Jing, 369 in the *Bencao Shiyi* of Chen Cangqi, 111 in the *Kaibao Bencao*, but only eight in the *Zhenglei Bencao* of Tang Shenwei and three in the *Bencao*

Yanyi Buyi of Zhu Zhenheng.[23] Li introduced a total of 374 new
drugs in his materia medica, drawing on a variety of sources,
particularly those of popular tradition. Such is the case with the
'knife-bean' (*daodu; Canavalia gladiata*), a leguminous plant that Li
noted was widely used and which had received no mention in any
materia medica, and the pseudo-ginseng, the celebrated *sanqi* (*Panax
notoginseng*). Other new drugs listed included a kind of gourd
known as *sigualuo* (*Luffa cylindrica*), which originated from India
and, according to Li Shizhen, was unknown before the Tang
dynasty; the *tianshili*, or 'chestnut of the lord of heaven' (*Aesculus
wilsonii*); the *maqianzi* (*Strychos nux-vomica*); and the *xiangsizi*, or
'seed of love' (*Abrus precatorius*), a leguminous plant whose seeds
contain a toxic albumen, abrin. Jacques Roi writes, with regard to
the *Abrus precatorius*:

> In China the use of seeds was recommended to combat fever
> and malevolent spirits. The remedy was as follows: when the
> patient hears the malevolent spirit, or when his ears buzz, take
> a seed from the *Abrus precatorius*, a seed from the castor-oil
> plant, and a seed from the *Croton tiglium*. Add a little cinnabar
> and beeswax. Grind them together to form a pill the size of a
> hemp-seed. Place cinders around the patient and light a small
> fire. The patient must then be made to vomit in the fire. As
> soon as the fire has consumed the vomit, a sign is made over
> the fire and the spirit dies.[24]

How were drugs classified in the *Bencao Gangmu*? A review of
previous classifications will enable us to appreciate Li Shizhen's
contribution. The *Shen'nong Bencaojing* divided drugs by virtue of
their 'toxicity': superior drugs were those reputed to be 'non-
poisonous', in contrast to inferior drugs, which were 'very
poisonous', while intermediate drugs were those 'without poison' or
which contained 'some poison'. Tao Hongjing, who revised and
commented on the *Shen'nong Bencaojing*, classified drugs within
these three categories according to their origins: jade and stone,
plant, tree, insect, reptile, quadruped, fruit, vegetable and grain.
This somewhat arbitrary classification was slightly modified during
the Tang by the compilers of the *Xinxiu Bencao* (*Newly-revised
Materia Medica*), then, in the eleventh century, by Tang Shenwei,
whose *Zhenglei Bencao* (*Classified Materia Medica*) arranged drugs
under the headings of jade and stone, plant, tree, products of
human origin, quadruped, bird, insect, reptile, fish, fruit, grain,
cereal and vegetable. Li Shizhen, in his *Bencao Gangmu*, used the
headings of water, fire, earth, metals and stone, plant, cereal,
vegetable, fruit, tree, products derived from 'garments and tools',

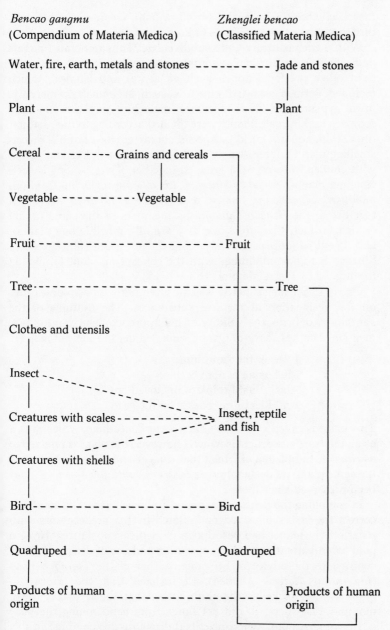

FIGURE 8.1 A comparison of Li Shizhen's classification of materia medica with that of Tang Shenwei. From *Li Shizhen Yanjiu* (Guangzhou: Guangdong Keji Chubanshe, 1984), p. 67.

insect, creatures with scales (reptiles, fish), creatures with shells, bird, quadruped and products of human origin.

Within each category were subdivisions. Thus minerals ('metals and stone' in Li Shizhen's words) were divided into metals, jade (and other precious stones such as agate) and 'stones', which included various assorted minerals such as cinnabar, mercury, mica, gypsum, steatite (soapstone), malachite, naphtha and even ordinary cooking salt. Plants were divided according to their habitat (mountain, aquatic, rock) or special character (for example, sweet-smelling plants). Interestingly, within the same subdivision, plants with similar features were grouped together. Thus, among 'sweet-smelling plants', *Angelica sinensis, Ligusticum wallichii, Cnidium monnieri, Ligusticum sinense* and *Angelica dahurica* are listed together in the *Bencao Gangmu* as members of the same family (which, in fact, they are since they are all umbelliferous plants), leaving one to suppose that, even if he did not specifically say so, Li Shizhen was not unfamiliar with the concept of 'plant family' as formulated by Pierre Magnol (1637–1715).

One of Li Shizhen's merits was his attempt to impose some order on the designation of medical substances. The example of the xanthium confirms the validity of his approach. The xanthium is mentioned in the *Classic of Odes* (*Shijing*) under the name of *juan'er*:

> I gather the xanthium,
> My basket is not yet filled.
> Alas! Alas! I think of my loved one
> And I leave my basket on the road . . .[25]

This plant is called *xi'er* in the *Shen'nong Bencaojing*, which lists it as an intermediate drug; elsewhere, however, the plant is referred to as *cang'er*. Li Shizhen affirmed that *cang'er* and *xi'er* were one and the same plant. Its designation as *cang'er* (*Xanthium sibiricum*) has been preserved since then.

In compiling the *Bencao Gangmu*, Li Shizhen generally sought to correct the errors inherited or initiated by his predecessors with regard to the names and description of medical substances. He also paid careful attention to the preparation and use of drugs. Thus, in contrast to the advice of Su Song, author of the *Tujing Bencao* (*Illustrated Materia Medica*), Li insisted that the eriocaulon (*gujingcao*) be picked in the ninth, rather than the second or third, month.[26] Elsewhere, Li did not flinch from condemning the false advice of charlatans who prescribed drugs to 'prolong life'. In Li's view, to believe, for example, that a mushroom such as the *lingzhi* (*Ganoderma lucidum*) could enable a person to avoid death was

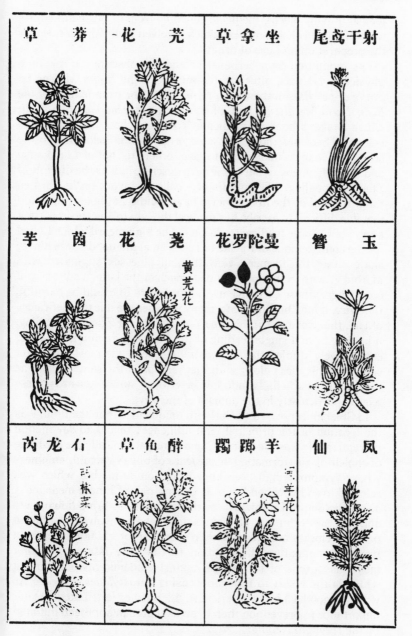

FIGURE 8.2   An illustration from the *Bencao Gangmu*. From *Bencao Gangmu* (Beijing: Renmin Weisheng Chubanshe, 1977).

foolish. Finally, herbal medicine benefited from Li Shizhen's efforts
to codify medical substances, which involved laying down rules for
the preparation and use of drugs.

Li's reputation as a herbalist should not obscure his role as a
physician. He was, after all, the author of the *Binhu Maixue* (*A
Study of the Pulse*), the *Qijing Bamai Kao* (*An Examination of the
Eight Extra Meridians*) and, of course, the *Bencao Gangmu* itself,
which is also a book on medicine. To what school did Li Shizhen
belong? There are those who categorise him as belonging to the
school of Zhang Yuansu and Li Gao, others to that of Liu Wansu
and Zhu Zhenheng, while some even describe him as the disciple of
Zhang Zhongjing. The authors of a collective work on Li Shizhen
think that all of the above views have validity, although they add
that it is difficult to ascribe Li's medical thought to any one important
strand of Chinese medical tradition.[27] The high regard which Li had
for the contributions of Li Gao or Liu Wansu did not dispose him to
share either the former's view that all illnesses originated with
morbid growth in the spleen and stomach or the latter's advocacy of
cold drugs, whose excessive use, according to Li, could be harmful.
Likewise, if for Zhu Zhenheng 'many illnesses are due to a deficiency
of *yin*', this was not Li Shizhen's opinion. As for Zhang Zhongjing,
it is clear from a single reading of the *Bencao Gangmu* that Li had
exhaustively studied the *Shanghanlun*, one of the most important
sources of his ideas along with the *Neijing*. At the same time, if he
thought it justified, Li adopted a critical stance towards these
works, particularly in the domain of therapy.

Li Shizhen expressed the hitherto unique idea that 'the brain was
the location of the principal vital influence', that is to say mental
perception. He was the first in China to reveal clinically the existence
of cholelithiasis (formation or presence of biliary calculi), an illness
whose symptoms had been known for some time but which was
referred to as hypochondria or epigastric pain. Chinese medicine is
also beholden to Li Shizhen for the use of ice to bring down fever
and for the technique of disinfection, which involved soaking a
patient's clothes in a steam bath in order to protect family members
from contamination. In addition to this, the *Bencao Gangmu*
mentions dozens of safeguards against epidemic disease, among
which is the resort to fumigation using *Atractylodes lancea*.[28] As
with all good Chinese physicians, Li Shizhen attributed greater
importance to prevention than to actual cure, an approach initiated
by the *Huangdi Neijing*:

> To wait for the illness to form
> before curing it,
> And for disorder to become evident
> before attending to it,
> Is like waiting to be thirsty
> Before sinking a well,
> Or to wait for war before
> Forging weapons.
> Is not this too late?[29]

It should also not be surprising to discover that the *Bencao Gangmu* includes a great many (more than 500) remedies to 'strengthen the body' and 'enhance life'. More than fifty of these remedies, moreover, were devised in the course of Li Shizhen's own medical experiments. In addition to ointments, pills and powders, Li recommended boiled broth of all kinds: wheat, rice, chestnut, tuber, radish, ginger and animal liver.

Pharmacognosist, pharmacologist and physician, but also a botanist, zoologist and mineralogist, Li Shizhen bequeathed to posterity a scientific body of work of the highest order. He was also a humanist who promoted Confucian-inspired medical ethics that called on everyone (including physicians) to care for their neighbour. Li's popularity has survived to the present, and the image of him observing the flower of the *Datura* is one of the most familiar to all Chinese.

Notes

1. Jacques Gernet, *A History of Chinese Civilization*, op. cit., p 391.
2. Yao Xueyin, *Li Zicheng* (Beijing: Zhongguo Oingnian Chubanshe, 1976/1977).
3. Yves Raguin, 'Un example d'inculturation: Matteo Ricci', *Lumen Vitae*, 39:3 (1984).
4. Jacques Gernet, *China and the Christian Impact* (Cambridge: Cambridge University Press, 1985), p 59.
5. L. Gallagher, *China in the Sixteenth Century: The Journals of Mathew Ricci* (New York: Random House, 1953), p 16.
6. Ibid., p 32.
7. Ibid., p 32.
8. Ibid.
9. *Yongle Dadian Yiyaoji* (Beijing: Renmin Weisheng Chubanshe, 1986).
10. Catherine Despeux, op. cit., p 31. Ming Wong, *Shanghanlun*, op. cit., p 64, translates *wenbing* (*wen* 'warm'; *bing* 'illness') as 'febrile illness'. *The Chinese-English Glossary of Common Terms in Traditional Chinese Medicine* (Guangzhou: Guangdong Keji Chubanshe, 1982) translates the term as 'seasonal febrile diseases'.

11. Fan Xingzhun, *Zhongguo Yixue Shilue* (Beijing: Zhongyi Guji Chubanshe, 1986), p 221.

12. Dai Sigong, *Tuiqiu Shiyi* (Nanjing: Jiangsu Kexue Jishu Chubanshe, 1984), p 22.

13. *Neike Zhaiyao* (Nanjing: Jiangsu Kexue Jishu Chubanshe, 1985), pp 41, 42. On its present use in traditional Chinese medicine, see *Zhongyixue Jichu*, op. cit., p 249: 'This remedy increases energy, invigorates the blood, fortifies the spleen and sustains the heart'.

14. Drawn from the *Piweilun* (*Treatise on the Spleen and Stomach*) by Li Gao (of whom Xue Ji was in some sense the heir), the 'decoction to invigorate the middle burner and enhance energy' was composed of *Astragalus membranaceus, Panax ginseng* (replaced today by *Codonopsis pilosula*), *Atractylodes macrocephela, Angelica sinensis, Bupleurum chinense, Cimicifuga foetida, Citrus reticulata* and *Glycyrrhiza uralensis*. According to the *Zhongyixue Jichu*, op. cit., p 246, this remedy 'increases energy, augments *yang*, and regularises and invigorates the spleen and liver'.

15. *Neike Zhaiyao*, op. cit., p 52.

16. Ibid., p 58. The 'decoction of hare's-ear', mentioned for the first time in the *Shanghanlun*, was composed of *Bupleurum chinense, Scutellaria baicalensis, Pinellia ternata, Zingiber officinale, Panax ginseng* (replaced today by *Codonopsis pilosula*), *Glycyrrhiza uralensis* and *Ziziphus jujuba*. On its use by Zhang Zhongjing, see Catherine Despeux, op. cit., p 64, and on its current use see *Zhongyixue Jichu*, op. cit., p 217.

17. The 'pill of eight ingredients', also known as the 'pill to invigorate the loins from the Golden Chest', is described today as being able to 'warm up and invigorate the *yang* of the loins'. It is composed, among other ingredients, of *Rehmannia glutinosa, Dioscorea opposita* and *Cornus officinalis*, as well as *Aconitum carmichaeli* and *Cinnamomum cassia*. It is often used in traditional Chinese medicine to treat nephritis, hypothyroidism and diabetes, which are considered the result of a lack of *yang* in the loins. The 'pill of six ingredients', which is not composed of either *Aconitum carmichaeli* or *Cinnamomum cassia* (considered tonics to enhance *yang*), is described as being able to 'sustain and invigorate the *yin* of the loins'. See *Zhongyixue Jichu*, op. cit., pp 250, 251.

18. Robert van Gulik, *Sexual Life in Ancient China*, op. cit., p 311.

19. The *Summary of Chinese Acupuncture*, op. cit., p 182, gives the following symptoms: 'sciatica, paralysis of the lower limb, painful hip-joints and periarticular tissue'.

20. I have been unable to consult the *Waike Zhengzong* by Chen Shigong, or the *Zhengzhi Zhunsheng* by Wang Kentang, and therefore draw on Fu Weikang, 'Ancient Physician's Concept of Tumours', *Traditional Chinese Medicine and Pharmacology*, op. cit., pp 96, 97, for the descriptions of cancer of the lip and breast.

21. *Hanshi Yitong* (Nanjing: Jiangsu Kexue Jishu Chubanshe, 1985).

22. Qian Yuanming, *Li Shizhen Yanjiu* (*Research on Li Shizhen*) (Guangzhou: Guangzhou Keji Chubanshe, 1984, p 17).

23. Ibid., pp 39, 40.

24. Jacques Roi, *Traité des Plantes Médicinales Chinoises*, op. cit., p 171.

25. *Le Livre des Poèmes* (*Classic of Odes*) (Paris: Albédo, 1986).

26. *Bencao Gangmu* (Beijing: Renmin Weisheng Chubanshe, 1977), 2:1105. This plant was especially used in ophthalmology, and traditional Chinese medicine today uses it in particular to treat nyctalopia.

27. *Li Shizen Yanjiu,* op. cit., p 132. This view is shared by Chen Ruquan, 'Bencao gangmu yixue xueshu sixiang' (Medical thought of the *Bencao gangmu*), *Zhonghua Yishi Zazhi,* no 1 (1987), pp 42–5.

28. As Jacques Léonard, *Archives du Corps: La Santé au Dix-neuvième siècle* (Paris: Ouest-France, 1986), p 81, notes: 'The methods of disinfection in the past certainly did not lack variety'. He adds: 'To prevent epidemic diseases, people placed aromatic substances like resin, incense and vinegar over live coals or on a red-hot iron shovel. Fir-cones, rosemary buds, and juniper-tree berries were also burnt in the same way.'

29. *Assaisonner les Esprits,* op. cit., p 43.

— 9 —

The Qing, from the Manchu Invasion of 1644 to the First Opium War, 1839–42

1644

Jacques Gernet notes that 'the Manchus settled in China like a race of lords destined to reign over a population of slaves'.[1] The imposition of the queue on the Chinese might not seem a significant example of Manchu overlordship until one realises that failure to wear the queue was a capital offence. The Manchus, however, had to deal with a Ming resistance movement in the south until 1661 and then from 1674–81 with a rebellion incited by the generals who had helped conquer south China. With this rebellion suppressed, Qing China entered a period of prosperity during the reigns of Kangxi (1662–1722), Yongzheng (1723–35) and Qianlong (1736–96). In 1895, Yan Fu (1853–1921), whose writings exercised a profound influence on Chinese thought, declared in one of his essays that a new Kangxi was needed to save China:

> He presided over the most glorious period of the dynasty; eminent ministers and generals were to be found at court. Better than anyone, he knew how to govern without causing disturbance and he presided over a peaceful and harmonious order. Yet no-one since antiquity had worked more enthusiastically in acquainting himself with the practical realities of life in China.[2]

Anxious to obtain the support of the scholar-literati class – some of them, such as Wang Fuzhi (1619–92) or Gu Yanwu (1613–82), had not hesitated in joining the resistance against the Manchus – the emperors of the eighteenth century encouraged intellectual life with state patronage of vast encyclopaedic enterprises that covered not only history and the sciences but also literature. This intellectual activity, however, was blighted by a rigorous censorship of which the notorious 'literary inquisition' marking the end of Qianlong's reign was the culmination. The puritanism of the new dynasty notwithstanding, a more varied literature emerged during this

130

period: the supernatural with Pu Songling's *Liaozhai Zhiyi* (*Strange Stories from an Eccentric's Studio*), the satirical with Wu Jingzi's *Rulin Waishi* (*The Scholars*), and the wistful with Cao Xueqin's *Honglou Meng* (*Dream of the Red Chamber*).

At the beginning of the nineteenth century, confidence gave way to anxiety in the face of an increasingly troublesome political, social and economic situation. Population growth (410 million by 1839) and natural calamities, in conjunction with a crisis of authority, encouraged secret-society-led peasant rebellion. However, as Jean Chesneaux notes, 'they were no more than dispersed and marginal expressions of peasant discontent, and gave way, between 1850–1870, to a major wave of peasant rebellions of exceptional size'.[3] It was against this background that commercial and political pressure from the western powers became more intense. The growth of the illegal opium trade led the imperial authorities to adopt strict measures in 1839 against traffickers and consumers, which were to culminate in the first Opium War and the Treaty of Nanjing in 1842.

The Chinese and their Physicians in the Eighteenth Century

The physicians were called in to treat him, but some said he was over-agitated and suffered from an excess of phlegm, some said he should exhale, some said he needed a warm sedative, while others even argued that seeing he was old he needed to take a tonic; each was so set in his own opinion that no-one could agree on a diagnosis.[4]

Molière himself would not have disowned these lines from the Chinese novel *Rulin Waishi* (*An Unofficial History of the Literati*), especially in light of his play *Le Malade Imaginaire* (*The Hypochondriac*), in which Béralde says of physicians: 'All the excellence of their art consists in the utterance of pompous nonsense and specious prattle that offers mere words in place of judgment and promises in place of results'. The author of *Rulin Waishi*, written in the mid-eighteenth century, extends the irony by having the reader go to the following chapter in order to discover the fate of the ailing old man, a traditional narrative technique whereby the denouement of an episode is suspended at the end of a chapter.

This important classical Chinese novel, in which the action begins at the end of the fifteenth century and concludes at the beginning of the seventeenth century, contains detailed medical references, even to the point of providing remedies. Thus in chapter 11 a certain Chen Hefu, after examining the pulse of a patient, remarks: 'Your pulse is rather feeble. The lungs control the breath, and the weakness of the pulse shows that you have a little phlegm.' Then he adds: 'I have observed that physicians nowadays often consider pinellia (*banxia*) rather hot; thus when they treat cases of phlegm they use hermodactyl (*beimu*). Actually, hermodactyl is not efficacious in cases of phlegm.' Chen Hefu therefore recommends for the patient a decoction of the 'four masters', to be taken with another decoction known as *erchen*: 'Take it warm before a meal. Two or three doses only are required. This will ease your kidneys so that the fiery humour does not rise easily, and then the illness will be cured.'[5] The conclusion of this episode reveals that the patient gradually recovers, which is not the case with the impecunious student who 'did not want to spend money on buying ginseng' so that 'after mid-autumn the physicians stopped prescribing medicine for him.'[6] The fate of the unfortunate young man is left to the imagination of the reader, but it is evident that ginseng was not cheap at that time. It was expensive enough to arouse a scholar's anger against a boatman who had eaten his 'walnut wafers': 'You dog! I've spent several hundreds of silver taels to have this medicine prepared; it has ginseng in it . . . You wretched cur, you've caused me a lot of expense!'[7] In a letter dated 12 April 1771, the Jesuit Jartoux wrote that ginseng 'was far too expensive for the man in the street'.[8]

The *Rulin Waishi* relates an episode in which a physician is accused of poisoning his patient because the latter had thrown himself into a river and drowned. The physician, interrogated by the magistrate looking into the case, replies:

> He had caught a chill, so I prescribed a medicine to make him sweat . . . the medicine contained eight drachms of *asarum*. There was a relative there at the time – a squat and round-faced fellow – who said that three drachms of *asarum* would prove fatal. But that is certainly not what the *Shen'nong Bencaojing* says . . . You can certainly analyse all the properties medicines have, but you will not be able to find a single medicine that will make people jump into the river!

The charges against the physician are dropped; moreover, the magistrate concludes that 'a physician is a benefactor, he would cut flesh from his own thigh in order to nourish and cure a seriously ill patient'.[9]

Chinese and European Medicine

The Jesuit missionary de Fontaney reported in a letter dated 15 February 1703 that the Kangxi emperor was particularly interested in the 'medicinal paste' that Louis XIV 'distributed among the poor throughout his kingdom. We informed the emperor of all the illnesses that such paste cured in France, and repeated demonstrations allowed the emperor to see for himself how it effected such a miraculous and rapid cure that a man on the verge of death was often out of danger the following day.' Kangxi himself fell ill but, continued de Fontaney, 'the Chinese physicians did not advise him to take this paste, and treated him in their own way; however, the emperor, feeling he was getting worse and fearing he might have a stroke, made up his own mind and ordered that he be given a half-measure of this paste. The fever subsided in the evening and in the following days he recovered . . .'. Subsequently, when the emperor suffered from a 'third attack of fever', de Fontaney recommended he take quinquina. 'He was expecting to suffer an attack that day at three in the afternoon, but it never came. He rested peacefully the rest of the day and during the night.'[10] It should be remembered that quinquina (the bark of several species of cinchona, yielding quinine and other febrifugal alkaloids) was then a fashionable medicine in France. La Fontaine praised its merits in his poem 'On Quinquina' (1682):

> Double, if there is need, the use of the bark,
> In accordance with the patient's strength.

Pierre Delaveau points out in his *Histoire et Renouveau des Plantes Medicinales* (*A History and Revival of Medicinal Plants*) that La Fontaine's poem was 'virtually a eulogy in praise of this efficacious bark, but also of Nature and Louis XIV, whose authority and financial encouragement (as La Fontaine was aware) enabled it to be adopted as a new medicine'.[11] In 1765, Zhao Xuemin included quinquina among the drugs listed in his *Bencao Gangmu Shiyi* (*Supplement to the* Bencao Gangmu).

On the other hand, another Jesuit, Dominique Parrenin (1665–1741), who enjoyed considerable prestige while he was in China from 1698 until his death, failed in his attempt to introduce western anatomy despite the interest of Kangxi, with whom Parrenin met frequently. However, Parrenin's scientific correspondence with the Paris Academy of Sciences, the Academy of Inscriptions and Letters and the St Petersburg Academy of Sciences stimulated a certain curiosity among his readers vis-à-vis Chinese medicine. He was able to inform eminent French scholars such as Fontanelle, Jean-Jacques Dortous de Mairan and Nicolas Fréret of various aspects of Chinese medicine. Samples of *Cordyceps sinensis* and *Angelica sinensis* that Parrenin sent from China were the first to be introduced to Europe. Moreover, such plant samples 'were the object of a research report by Réamur read to the Academy of Sciences in 1726'.[12]

Réamur's 'Dissertation sur l'origine, la dénomination, la nature et la curation des maladies vénériennes à la Chine' (Dissertation on the origins, designation, nature and cure of venereal disease in China) was appended to Jean Astruc's French translation of *De Morbis Venereis* (*Treatise on Venereal Disease*) in 1743. On 11 August 1730, Parrenin wrote to Dortous de Mairan:

> When I hear Chinese physicians speak on the principles of illness, I do not detect any accuracy or validity in their arguments; but when they apply to their patients remedies they have devised through taking the pulse and examining different parts of the head, I see that such remedies practically always have a beneficial effect.[13]

Voltaire, who was aware of Parrenin's correspondence, echoed the same view in his *Essai sur les Mœurs*: 'Medical theory among the Chinese is still based on ignorance and error; however, Chinese physicians practise quite successfully'. In any event, remarked the Jesuit, d'Entrecolles, in a letter dated 11 May 1726, 'knowledge of diseases and their cures has not been as backward in China as it has, perhaps, in Europe, where some have dismissed Chinese physicians as unlearned or fakesters'. D'Entrecolles added, with regard to treatises on Chinese medicine, that 'if they had been translated into our language, European physicians would have welcomed what they had to say on the different kinds of illness, their diagnoses and symptoms, as well as on their remedies and effects'.[14]

Books on Medicine

China in the eighteenth century witnessed a boom in encyclopaedias. Collections of all kinds flourished, among which was the vast encyclopaedia of 10,000 chapters by Chen Menglei, the *Gujin Tushu Jicheng* (*Collection of Ancient and Modern Works*), which has considerable interest for the history of Chinese medicine. Of this work, which was published in 1726, 520 chapters concern medicine. The most famous medical work of this kind, however, is undoubtedly the *Yizong Jinjian* (*Golden Mirror of Medicine*) by Wu Qian; 250 years after its publication (1742), it still remains an important reference work. Mention should also be made of the anthology completed in 1782 and known as the *Siku Quanshu* (*Complete Writings of the Four Treasuries*), a collection of books divided into four sections (classics, history, philosophy, miscellanea). Included in the collection are a large number of medical works. One of the scholars associated with this particular encyclopaedic enterprise was Dai Zhen (1723–77), a key figure in the world of Chinese science during the Qing.

Encyclopaedic works on medicine also included collections of works by the same author, which were virtually medical compendia because of the broad variety of topics covered. The earliest such collection comprised the seven works of Zhang Lu (1617–1700), whose *Zhangshi Yitong* (*A Summary of Master Zhang's Medical Thought*), written towards the end of his life, revealed an affinity with the 'school of warming and invigoration' (*wenbu*) that had developed during the Ming. An opponent of this school was Xu Dachun, alias Xu Lingtai (1693–1771), whose *Xu Lingtai Yixue Quanshu* (*Complete Medical Works of Xu Lingtai*) comprised seventeen volumes. Xu demonstrated an attachment to the medical values of the past, and in his *Yixue Yuanliulun* (*The Origin and Development of Medicine*), published in 1757, he pleaded for a return to the sources: 'Words must be based on the classical writings, and treatment must conform with ancient methods'. He thus recommended that in order to regain strength after illness one had to be content, like the ancients, with eating the five cereals (e.g. rice, millet) rather than taking fortifying drugs. He adopted a similar approach in the *Yiguan Bian*, a critique of the *Yiguan* by Zhao Xianke, one of the followers of the *wenbu* school. Xu considered the teachings of the *Shanghanlun* as a 'golden rule, and law set in jade', adding that 'One should not add or delete one single character'.

Besides the four works compiled at the beginning of the eighteenth century by Feng Zhaozhang, known as the *Fengshi Jinnang Milu* (*Secret Notes from Master Feng's Brocade Pouch*), and the ten books written by Huang Yuanyu, a physician influenced by the seventeenth-century follower of the *wenbu* school, Zhang Jiebin, mention should be made of the seven works by Shen Jin'ao (1717–76), published in 1773 under the general title of *Shenshi Zunshengshu* (*Master Shen's Books on Respect for Life*), and the sixteen works of Chen Xiuyuan (1753–1823), which popularised medicine among a wider audience.

At the same time, more modest publications on medicine appeared. They tended to be introductions, such as the *Yixue Xinwu* (*An Understanding of Medicine*) published in 1732 by Cheng Guopeng. Cheng discussed the four methods of examination (observation, listening, interrogating the patient, and pulsing), the eight leading principles (external, internal, cold, hot, empty, full, *yin* and *yang*) and the seven therapeutic techniques (sweating, induced vomiting, purging, harmonisation, warming, purification and dispersal) that all served as the basis of medical training. Medical instruction at this time was essentially passed from father to son or from master to disciple.

The *Zhengzhi Huibu* by Li Yongcui, which dates from 1687, is entirely devoted to illnesses relying on internal medicine for treatment, as well as to their symptoms. Since the author also provides therapeutic tips, the book is a virtual mini-encyclopaedia of medicine. The *Yibian* (1751) by He Mengyao also aimed to be as practical, likewise the *Bencao Beiyao* (*Emergency Materia Medica*) compiled in 1694 by Wang Ang (discussed below as a commentator on the *Huangdi Neijing*). Wu Yiluo (Wu Zuncheng) in 1757 added to Wang Ang's work with the *Bencao Congxin*, which listed 721 drugs (as opposed to 470 in the *Bencao Beiyao*). The *Bencao Congxin* mentions for the first time the root of *Panax quinquefolium*, known popularly as 'Canton ginseng', although its formal Chinese name, *xiyangsheng* ('Panax from the West'), indicates a more distant origin. Other introductory works included the *Bihua Yijing* (*Bihua's Mirror of Medicine*), published in 1824 by Jiang Hantun, alias Jiang Bihua (Jiang 'who writes of flowers').

Commentators on the *Huangdi Neijing*

The *Huangdi Neijing*, the 'bible' of Chinese medicine, continued to arouse the interest of commentators from the end of the seventeenth century to the beginning of the nineteenth century. Such commentators were following in the footsteps of Ma Shi, Wu Kun, Zhang Jiebin and Li Zhongzi, all of whose works (published during the Ming) were reissued during the Qing period.

Zhang Jiebin's idea of classifying the contents of the *Huangdi Neijing* under specific headings attracted commentators such as Wang Ang (b. 1615), who compiled an annotated edition of the *Suwen* and *Lingshu*. In addition to this commentary, published under the title of *Suwen Lingshu Leizhuan Yuezhu*, Wang wrote a materia medica (mentioned above) and various remedy books. Chen Xiuyuan adopted a similar approach, regrouping the two sections of the *Huangdi Neijing* to compile his *Lingsu Jizhu Jieyao*, one of his sixteen volumes on medicine. Thus, for example, under the heading 'Looking at the facial complexion' – one of the procedures of traditional diagnosis – the *Lingsu Jizhu Jieyao* has extracts from various chapters of the *Huangdi Neijing* interspersed with the commentator's notes (with a different print).

One of the most important annotated editions of the *Huangdi*

Neijing at this time is the *Huangdi Neijing Suwen Lingshu Jizhu*, produced by Zhang Zhicong in 1672. Zhang's pupil, Gao Shishi, continued the enterprise with the *Huangdi Suwen Zhijie* (*A Correct Explanation of the* Suwen), composed in 1695. Huang Yuanyu, mentioned earlier, was also interested in the *Suwen*; his *Suwen Xuanjie* (*Explanation of the* Suwen) dates from 1756.

The *Shanghanlun*, a 'Best Seller'

Far from fading, the *Shanghanlun*'s time-honoured reputation grew during the Qing period. Numerous works, in fact, were written on Zhang Zhongjing's famous treatise on *shanghan* illnesses. In addition to the *Shanghanlun* by Zhang Suichen, alias Zhang Qingzi (1589–1668), and the *Shanghanlun Zhijie* (*Correct Explanation of the* Shanghanlun) by Zhang Lingshao – one of the 'three Zhangs' of Quantang (present-day Hangzhou) along with Zhang Suichen and Zhang Zhicong – there were works by Yu Chang, Ke Qin, Xu Dachen and You Yi. Yu Chang (1585–1664), whose *Shanghanlun-pian* (published in 1648) refers especially to the *Shanghanlun Tiaobian* of his Ming colleague, Fang Youzhi, was particularly interested in illnesses of the *taiyang* meridian, one of the six syndromes described by Zhang Zhongjing. For his part, Ke Qin (1662–1735) included his observations on the *Shanghanlun* in three volumes, under the title *Shanghan Laisuji*, while Xu Dachun applied himself in 1759 to compiling the *Shanghanlun Leifang* (*Classified Remedies of the* Shanghanlun). You Yi (d. 1749) is known for his *Shanghan Guanzhuji*, a collection known as a 'thread of pearls' because of its layout, which was not published until 1810. Other devotees of the *Shanghanlun* at this time included Zhou Yangjun and Chen Yaodao. Zhou Yangjun at the end of the seventeenth century contributed to the *Shanghanlun Sanzhu* (*The Three Commentaries on the* Shanghanlun), the other two being compiled by Fang Youzhi and Yu Chang. Chen Yaodao published in 1679 the *Shanghan Bianzheng* (*Distinctions among* Shanghan *illnesses*).

Another work by Zhang Zhongjing, the *Jingui Yaolue* (*Summary of the Golden Chest*), enjoyed considerable popularity during the Qing, and was the subject of various editions and commentaries. The authors of such commentaries were all devotees of the *Shanghanlun*: Zhou Yangjun, who published the *Jingui Fanglun Yanyi* (completed by Zhao Yide in 1368); You Yi, whose *Jingui Yaolue Xindian* appeared in 1732 and *Jinguiyi* in 1768; and Chen Nianzu (Chen Xiuyuan), who published not only a commentary on the *Jingui Yaolue* (*Jingui Yaolue Qianzhu*) in 1803 but also one on the *Shanghanlun* (*Shanghanlun Qianzhu*), of which several editions dating from the nineteenth century have survived.

Heat, the Origin of All Diseases

The notion of heat as a pathogenic agent had been formulated in the twelfth century by Liu Wansu, founder of the Hejian school. Liu's ideas, revived during the fourteenth century by Zhu Zhenheng, Wang Lu and Dai Sigong, culminated in the distinction being made between *shanghan* ('cold-induced illness') and *wenbing* (febrile illness). With Wu Youxing in the seventeenth century, this particular approach to pathogenesis was renewed with the theory of 'violent influences', which, by penetrating the body through the mouth and nose, spread *wenyi* (pestilence in the general sense of 'epidemics'). Wu's theory, as outlined in the *Weiyilun* (*On Pestilence*), exerted considerable influence on what is known as the 'school of febrile illness' (*wen[re]bing*, literally 'illnesses associated with heat'). The most significant representatives of this school included Ye Gui, Xue Xue, Zhou Yangjun, Dai Tianzhang, Yang Xuan, Wu Tang and Yu Lin.

After the *Weiyilun* by Wu Youxing, the *Wenrelun* (*On Febrile Illnesses*) by Ye Gui, alias Ye Tianshi (1667–1746), gave new prominence to the study of *wenbing*. For Ye Gui, most febrile illnesses were contracted through the respiratory organs. Pathogenic agents, referred to by the term *wenxie* ('harmful influences of heat'), 'attacked the lungs and contaminated the pericardium'. Moreover, Ye Gui distinguished four stages in the development of *wenbing*: *wei, qi, ying* and *xue*, which respectively corresponded to an appropriate therapy. Xue Xue (1681–1770), a contemporary of Ye Gui, likewise focused on the analysis and treatment of febrile illnesses; his *Shire Tiaobian* discussed 'illnesses associated with heat and humidity'. Zhou Yangjun, like Xue Xue a native of Suzhou (the 'Venice of China'), in addition to writing commentaries on the *Shanghanlun* and the *Jingui Yaolue*, wrote the *Wenreshuyi Quanshu* (*Complete Work on Heat-induced Illnesses*). In this work, Zhou distinguished between *wenbing* ('illnesses associated with warmth'), *rebing* ('illnesses associated with extreme heat') and *yibing* (epidemic diseases), among which was an affliction known as 'swollen head' (*datou*), characterised by tumefaction and a flushed complexion. Dai Tianzhang, in his *Guangwenyilun* (*On Pestilence*), composed around 1722, showed how *wenyi* differed from *shanghan*. His colleague, Zhou Yangjun, noted that *shanghan* developed 'from the

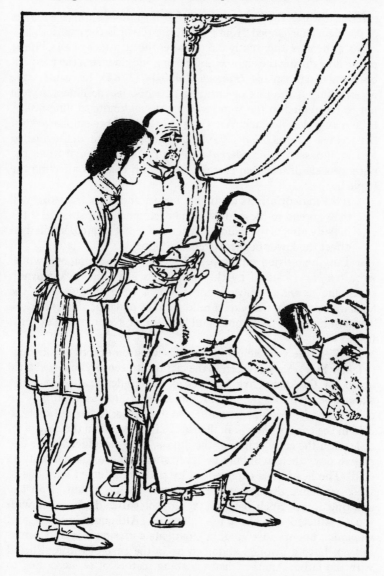

FIGURE 9.1   Ye Tianshi. From *Zhongguo Gudai Yixuejia De Gushi* (Shanghai: Shaonian Ertong Chubanshe, 1979).

exterior towards the interior', while febrile illnesses and other types of pestilence developed 'from the interior towards the exterior'.

Such theories apparently did not alter the attitudes of all Chinese physicians during the eighteenth century, judging from the need felt by Yang Xuan, in his *Hanwen Tiaobian* (1784), to reassert the notion that, at the risk of harming patients, febrile illnesses were not to be treated in the same way as for cold-induced illnesses. A little over a decade later, Wu Tang (1758–1836) re-emphasised in his treatise on *wenbing* (*Wenbing Tiaobian*) what distinguished febrile illnesses from *shanghan*, noting in particular that the pathogenesis of *wenbing* corresponded with changes affecting the triple burner:

> If the malady affects the higher burner and is not treated, it will then spread to the middle burner (stomach and spleen); if the malady affects the middle burner and is not treated, it will then affect the lower burner (liver and kidneys).

Wu Tang also listed nine types of febrile illnesses, among which were *fengwen*, caused by the wind; *wenre*, or the 'heat-warmth syndrome'; *wendu*, whose acute features were expressed by the term *du* ('poison'); *wennue*, a mild form of malaria; *shiwen*, or the 'warmth-humidity' syndrome; and *shuwen*, or syndrome of 'extreme heat'.

In 1794, the year he completed his work on eruptive epidemics (*Yizhen Yide*), Yu Lin (born in the eighteenth century) insisted once again on the distinctive features of *yi* (epidemic diseases) and *shanghan*, juxtaposing, for example, fever and susceptibility to cold. Fever, he explained, manifested itself prior to susceptibility to cold in the case of *shanghan* illness, and vice versa in the case of *yi*, at least in the early stages of the illness, since he added: 'After one or two days there will only be fever and no more susceptibility to cold'. The headaches experienced by patients afflicted with one of these epidemic diseases were compared to the action of an axe splitting wood. Such patients would not suffer deafness as with those afflicted by *shanghan* illnesses. Although both *yi* and *shanghan* might cause vomiting, patients suffering from the former did not have a swollen abdomen as in the case of those afflicted with the latter. Another distinguishing feature of *yi*, according to Yu Lin, was the appearance of cutaneous lesions known as *ban*, or *zhen*, whence came the term *yizhen* ('eruptive epidemic diseases').

Yu Lin described the symptoms of such diseases. 'At the beginning the patient's entire body is like ice. The complexion is of a dirty colour. The mouth is like it is full of frost. The head feels as if it is being split apart . . .' An 'enormous unquenchable thirst', 'never-ending pains in the stomach', the tongue 'as hard as iron, and as thick as armour plate' or 'covered with white spots like pearls', vomiting and constipation are also characteristic symptoms of these 'eruptive epidemic diseases', among which are included mumps and jaundice ('the whole body is like gold'). Incurable diseases are recognised by a combination of symptoms such as 'greenish facial complexion', 'a state of bewilderment', 'perspiration falling like rain', 'wanting to vomit but not being able to' and 'wanting to urinate but not being able to'. In less serious cases, however, the *Yizhen Yide* recommends a therapeutic method based on the following principle: 'Dissipate (*qing*: literally "to purify") the heat and neutralise the poison'. One of the most celebrated of Yu Lin's remedies used gypsum (*shigao*: 'stone plaster') as a base, mixed with various ingredients such as *Coptis chinensis, Gardenia jasminoides, Scutellaria baicalensis, Anemarrhena asphodeloides, Paeonia lactiflora, Scrophularia ningpoensis* and *Forsythia suspensa*.[15]

The New Anatomy

As previously mentioned, the attempt by Dominique Parrenin to introduce western anatomy to China came to naught. Chinese anatomy continued to rely essentially on the information provided in the *Huangdi Neijing*, to which little had been added since its completion. In 1830, Wang Qingren (1768–1831), in his *Yilin Gaicuo* (*Errors Corrected from the Forest of Physicians*), sought to correct the misconceptions handed down by tradition, for example the idea that 'urine originated from excrement' or the assumption that 'there were twenty-four holes in the lung'. Moreover, his observations of corpses abandoned in public cemeteries and execution grounds led him to discover the abdominal aorta, the vena cava, the pyloric sphincter ('which obstructed the path to the alimentary canal' in Wang Qingren's words), the hepatic duct, the pancreas and the diaphragm, which Wang described as 'thin as paper'. He also established that it was the brain, and not the heart, that controlled thought and memory. The poor conditions under which Wang carried out his research, however, inevitably led to some erroneous assumptions.

Gynaecologists, Paediatricians, Massage Therapists, Dermatologists and Other Specialists

The most important gynaecologist at the beginning of the Qing was without doubt Fu Shan, or Fu Qingzhu (1607–84). He was not yet forty in 1644 when the Ming dynasty fell. Out of loyalty to the Ming, Fu refused to collaborate with the Manchu invaders, despite

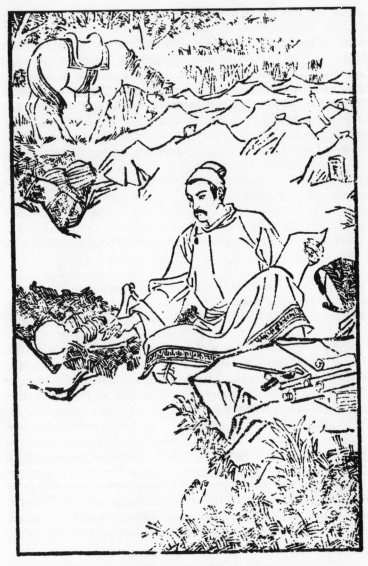

FIGURE 9.2   Wang Qingren. From *Zhongguo Gudai Yixuejia De Gushi* (Shanghai: Shaonian Ertong Chubanshe, 1979).

the emperor Kangxi's policy of enlisting the support of the scholar class. Fu Shan was a versatile scholar, noted writer, skilled calligrapher and celebrated physician. He is known especially as a gynaecologist and obstetrician, due to the corpus of his medical writings collected under the title of *Fu Qingzhu Nuke* (*Fu Qingzhu's Gynaecology*), which was not published until 1827. One work that circulated during Fu Shan's lifetime was the *Jiyin Gangmu* (*A Synopsis of Female Illnesses*) by Wu Zhiwang in 1620 that was completed and republished by a certain Wang Qi in 1665. In the very same year that Fu Shan died, his colleague Xiao Xun published a treatise on gynaecology, the *Nuke Jinglun*. During the eighteenth century, gynaecology and obstetrics were further enriched with the *Nuke Qieyao* (*Indispensable Aspects of Gynaecology*) by Wu Benli, published in 1773.

During the same period, paediatrics was the subject of two books, the *Youke Tiejing* (*Iron Mirror of Paediatrics*) by Xia Ding in 1695, and the *Youyou Jicheng* by Chen Xiazheng in 1750. Chen Xiazheng considered that 'the *zang* and *fu* organs of a small child were not completely formed' and that, as a result, they 'could not support a surfeit of medicine'. He thus championed external treatment such as massage, hot compresses and even hypnotism. He also made use of suppositories containing honey to stimulate the bowels, and did not hesitate in resorting to traditional popular remedies. One example of this was his use of purslane to combat dysentery. With regard to massage, a treatise on massage therapy was available from the beginning of the seventeenth century, the *Xiao'er Tuina Mizhi* (*Hidden Significance of Infant Massage*) by Gong Tingxian (Gong Yunlin), which was published several times. This work was complemented by the *Xiao'er Tuina Guangyi* by Xiong Yingxiong, a specialist in massage therapy at the beginning of the Qing.

Among the diseases afflicting the Chinese population during the seventeenth and eighteenth centuries were smallpox, to be discussed below, and malaria, which was the subject of a treatise at the beginning of the Qing by Lu Zhiyi, the *Jienue Lunshu*. There were also specialists in ophthalmology and laryngology. The year of the Manchu conquest (1644) witnessed the appearance of the *Shenshi Baohan* (*Precious Letter Concerning Vision*) by Fu Renyu, who, in addition to other therapeutic measures, made use of acupuncture and moxibustion. So too did the laryngologist Zheng Han, or Zheng Meijian (1721–87), whose *Chonglou Yuyao* was not published until the first half of the nineteenth century. The work notably contains a description of a disease akin to diphtheria ('white throat' in Chinese). In the fields of acupuncture and moxibustion, reference continued to be made to Yang Jizhou's *Zhenjiu Dacheng*, which was published in several editions between the end of the seventeenth century and the beginning of the nineteenth.

The most significant figures of external medicine were Qi Kun, Wang Weide, Gu Shicheng and Gao Bingjun. Qi Kun drained the pus from abscesses, employing a method similar to that of using a gauze tent. A description of the process is found in the *Waike Dacheng* (*The Great Successes of External Medicine*), which Qi Kun published in 1655 and which deals with all kinds of cutaneous ailments: abscesses, anthrax, wounds and even goitre. Three-quarters of a century later, there appeared the *Waike Zhengzhi Quanshengji*, a treatise by Wang Weide devoted to the diagnosis and treatment of illnesses requiring external medicine. His therapeutic approach was based on the principle of 'regarding dissolution, or dispersal (*xiao*), as the most valuable method, and only using one's hands with circumspection'. He thus opposed the unthinking use of surgical instruments. Wang was the father of celebrated remedies such as pills 'to stimulate dissolution'. His book has enjoyed considerable renown up to the present, since a number of the remedies which it prescribes are still used in traditional dermatology. Two other works from this period contributed to the development of this branch of medicine: the *Yangyi Daquan* (*Summary of Skin Specialists*), published in 1760, and the *Yangke Xindeji* (*Results of the Study of Skin Diseases*), published in 1805. The former, compiled by Gu Shicheng, is a collection of texts on 'skin diseases' (*yang*) in the broadest sense of the term. A whole chapter, for example, is devoted to the treatment of wounds caused by a fall or a blow. The book also gives information on how to react to a snake-bite and gives advice on emergency treatment. Finally, it describes a method of correcting hare-lip. On the other hand, the *Yangke Xindeji* by Gao Bingjun is, as its title indicates (*xinde*: 'what the mind reaps from the study'), reflections based on the author's personal experiences in the treatment of skin lesions.

Other works on external medicine include the *Dongtian Aozhi* (*Mysteries from the Immortals' Paradise*) by Chen Shiduo (1694) and two books on traumatology, the *Shangke Buyao* (1808) by Qian Changxiu and the *Shangke Huizuan* by Hu Tingguang, written in 1815 but preserved in its manuscript form until 1962.

The Use of the Smallpox Virus to Combat Smallpox

> Her son caught smallpox and ran a fever for a whole day; the doctor said this was a dangerous disease and used rhinoceros horn, gentian and cinders of burnt teeth to cure it. However, the rash did not come out as it should have done, and although the mother implored the gods and made prayers it was all to no purpose. After one week, the pale and plump little fellow died.[16]

This extract from the *Wailin Rushi* (*Unofficial History of the Literati*) says much about the traumas caused by smallpox, known poetically in Chinese as 'heavenly flowers' (*tianhua*). This is notwithstanding the fact that variolation was practised in China at this time. The Jesuit d'Entrecolles, in a letter dated 11 May 1726, described 'the Chinese method of obtaining the smallpox virus for the benefit of children', while informing his correspondent that it was not incumbent upon him 'to take sides for or against those who favoured the insertion of the smallpox virus'. This did not in any way prevent d'Entrecolles from emphasising that 'such a method was not new to China, since much thought had already gone into the several ways of perfecting it'.[17]

According to Yu Maokun, whose *Douke Jinjing Fujijie* was published in 1727, variolation had been practised in China since the years 1567–72. A detailed description of the process can be found in the *Zhangshi Yitong* (*Summary of Master Zhang's Medicine*), compiled in 1695, and in the *Yizong Jinjian* (*Golden Mirror of Medicine*), written in 1742. One of the methods consisted of extracting dry variolous scabs, reducing them to a fine powder and then having the patient inhale it through the nose with the aid of a silver tube. As for the risks involved in this kind of inoculation, one reads in a letter by d'Entrecolles, citing one of the three remedies communicated to him:

> When the powder has been inserted in the nose and a fever breaks out, if the pustules do not appear until the third day it is guaranteed that out of ten children eight or nine will be saved; but if the pustules appear on the second day, five out of ten children will be at considerable risk. Finally, if the pustules appear on the first day fever breaks out, not one of the ten children will be saved.[18]

Despite the imperfection of such a method, it is undeniable that variolation as practised in China played a significant role in the prevention of smallpox. Knowledge of the process quickly spread to Europe, not only in France (due primarily to the series of letters written by French Jesuits in China published under the title *Lettres Edifiantes et Curieuses de Chine*) but also in Russia. In a book dating from 1847, Yu Zhengxie noted: 'During the Kangxi reign, Russia sent people to China to study the cure of smallpox through vaccination'. Reference might also be made to the well-known story of the wife of the British ambassador to Turkey who at the beginning of the eighteenth century had her children vaccinated by the Chinese method.

Supplement to the *Bencao Gangmu*

Zhao Xuemin was happy to have been able to 'gather up' (*shi*) from the 'Garden of Cultivation' what Li Shizhen had 'lost' (*yi*) while compiling the *Bencao Gangmu* (*Materia Medica*). After forty years of research, Zhao Xuemin bequeathed to Chinese medicine and pharmacy a 'supplement' (*shiyi*: literally 'to gather up lost objects') to the *Bencao Gangmu*, known as the *Bencao Gangmu Shiyi*. A native of Hangzhou, where he was born at the beginning of the eighteenth century, the young Zhao Xuemin benefited from paternal concern for his future and that of his brother, his father arranging for them a place of study known as the 'Garden of Cultivation'. Zhao familiarised himself with the classics of medicine in the library and with medicinal plants in the garden. Although it was his younger brother whom Xuemin's father intended for a career in medicine, the interest shown by Xuemin in the natural sciences decided otherwise.

The *Bencao Gangmu Shiyi* was published in 1765. A total of 921 drugs were listed under the categories of water, fire, earth, metals, stones, herbs, trees, creeping plants, flowers, fruit, seeds, vegetables, utensils, birds, quadrupeds, creatures with scales or shells, and insects. Zhao's supplement included two new categories – creeping plants and flowers – while eliminating products of human origin listed in Li Shizhen's original *Materia Medica*. The most significant feature of Zhao's work, however, was the introduction of medical substances that Zhao doubtless had learnt to recognise and use while talking with itinerant physicians, whose long-standing experience he admired. For example, Zhao referred to an alga (seaweed) on the coasts of Fujian and Guangdong, *Caloglossa leprieurii*, which is effective in the treatment of ascariasis (threadworm). Among drugs of foreign origin listed were the bark of the *Cinchona ledgeriana* (the well-known quinquina) to treat malaria, and the seeds of the *Sterculla scaphigera* used to combat pharyngitis.[19]

Prior to the publication of his *Bencao Gangmu Shiyi*, Zhao

Xuemin had recorded in the *Chuanya* (1759) the teachings he had received from itinerant physicians (*chuanyi*: 'physicians who travel from one place to another'). The popularity of these physicians, also known as 'bell physicians' (*Lingyi*) because they announced their presence by means of a small bell, stemmed from the fact that they prescribed medicinal plants which were accessible and hence economic in price. This was the reason, in fact, why Zhao Xuemin thought highly of these physicians (it might be said that the famous 'barefoot doctors' of post-1949 China were their heirs), concluding that the drugs they recommended were 'cheap', 'efficient' and 'practical'. Zhao noted in the *Chuanya* that a drug need not be expensive, berating the medical quacks whose scientific skills did not match their high fees; such people, Zhao observed, knew how to prescribe an expensive tonic but did not know how to recognise a medicinal plant. Some writers of medical texts, in fact, laid down principles of medical ethics. Thus Zhang Lu, a physician of the seventeenth century, in his *Zhangshi Yitong* (*Summary of Master Zhang's Medicine*), specified 'ten prohibitions' to govern the physician's behaviour, such as not to 'go only one's way', not to 'be over-confident and act carelessly', and not to 'denigrate one's colleagues'.

Notes

1. Jacques Gernet, *A History of Chinese Civilization*, op. cit., p 465.
2. *Les Manifestes de Yen Fou*, translated from the Chinese and introduced by François Houang (Paris: Fayard, 1977). In 1898, Yan Fu translated T. Huxley's *Evolution and Ethics*.
3. Jean Chesneaux, *Peasant Revolts in China 1840–1949* (London: Thames and Hudson, 1973), p 23.
4. Wu Jingzi, *Chronique Indiscrète des Mandarins* (Unofficial History of the Literati). Translated from the Chinese by Tchang Fou-jouei, and introduced by André Lévy (Paris: Gallimard, 1976), 1:314. An English version of the novel is *The Scholars*, translated by Yang Hsien-yi and Gladys Yang (Beijing: Foreign Language Press, 1973). This translation has tended to follow the French version, since there are considerable differences between the two existing translations.
5. Ibid., p 171 (*The Scholars*, p 132). The Chinese term for pinella is *banxia*. The earliest reference to hermodactyl (*beimu*) is found in the *Shen'nong Bencaojing*. In his *Bencao Gangmu*, Li Shizhen gives a remedy of pills with *beimu* as a base to 'dissolve phlegm' (*hua tan*) and particularly emphasises the antitussient properties of this liliaceous plant. With Zhao Xuemin's *Bencao Gangmu Shiyi* (1765), a distinction was made between *chuanbeimu* (*Fritillaria cirrhosa*) and *zhebeimu* (*Fritillaria thunbergii*). The decoction of the 'four rulers', prescribed by Wang Ji to sustain the energy of his patients afflicted with syphilis, is here supplemented with ingredients used in the *erchen* decoction, principally

composed of *Pinella ternata*, a plant used for its antitussient and antiemetic effects.

6. Ibid., p 78 (*The Scholars*, p 63).
7. Ibid., p 91 (*The Scholars*, p 70).
8. *Lettres Edifiantes et Curieuses de Chine pas des Missionnaires Jésuites (1702–1776)* (Paris: Garnier-Flammarion, 1979), p 176.
9. *Chronique Indiscrète des Mandarins*, op. cit., p 352 (*The Scholars*, pp 266–7). *Asarum sieboldi* appears as one of the superior drugs in the *Shen'nong Bencaojing*, which recognised its benefits in soothing headaches. It is used today not only to cure headaches but also to treat rheumatic pain and toothache.
10. *Lettres Edifiantes*, op. cit., pp 133–6.
11. Pierre Delaveau, *Histoire et Renouveau des Plantes Médicinales* (Paris: Albin Michel, 1982), p 190.
12. Yvonne Grover, 'La correspondance scientifique du P. Dominique Parrenin', in *Les Rapports entre la Chine et l'Europe au Temps des Lumières* (Paris: Belles Lettres, 1980), p 87.
13. *Lettres Edifiantes*, op. cit., p 363.
14. *Lettres Edifiantes*, op. cit., p 341.
15. Yu Lin, *Yizhen Yide* (Nanjing: Jiangsu Kexue Jishu Chubanshe, 1985).
16. *Chronique Indiscrète des Mandarins*, op. cit., p 87 (*The Scholars*, p 67).
17. *Lettres Edifiantes*, op. cit., pp 331, 335, 341. D'Entrecolles was not mistaken in believing that the Chinese, in giving the name *dou* to variolous pustules, 'had in mind the shape of the pustules, which formed on the skin like peas'. The Chinese for 'pea' is, in fact, *dou*, while the character for smallpox (also *dou*) contains the character for 'pea'.
18. *Lettres Edifiantes*, op. cit., p 333.
19. The *Cinchona ledgeriana* has since been transplanted to Taiwan, Hainan island and Yunnan. The *Sterculia scaphigera* grows in Vietnam, Thailand and other South-east Asian countries (such as Indonesia) with whom China at the time had commercial relations.

10

The Qing,
1842–1911

From Empire to Republic

The treaties of 1842–4, signed with Britain, France and the United States, 'opened' the ports of Guangzhou, Shanghai, Ningbo, Xiamen (Amoy) and Fuzhou to foreign trade and residence, as well as granting foreigners in these treaty ports the right of extraterritoriality. Persistent demands for treaty-revision led to the second Opium War (1856–60), during which an Anglo-French expeditionary force occupied Beijing, looting and destroying the famed Summer Palace. In France, Victor Hugo angrily declared: 'Two bandits entered the Summer Palace one day. One looted it, the other set fire to it . . . in the judgment of history one of these two bandits will be known as France, the other as England'.[1]

At the same time, the Manchus were confronted with the Taiping rebellion, whose leader Hong Xiuquan (1814–64) 'believed to have found in the Bible an explanation for his visions which, he asserted, conferred on him a divine and liberating mission'.[2] Hong's God-worshippers' Society, organised in 1845, gained the support of the disadvantaged in Guangxi province with its egalitarian millenarianism. In 1850, the God-worshippers' Society resorted to open rebellion, and by 1853, after a series of military victories, had occupied Nanjing and made it the capital of the Heavenly Kingdom of Great Peace. The Taiping thrust towards Beijing, however, was repelled by imperial troops. From 1859, power in the Taiping capital passed into the hands of Hong Ren'gan, a reformer with pro-western sympathies. Nevertheless, growing corruption and division in the Taiping administration at Nanjing allowed the imperialist forces, assisted from 1860 onwards by the western powers, to take the offensive, and Nanjing was retaken by the Qing in 1864.

After the death of the Xianfeng Emperor in 1861, a joint regency was established under the empress-consort Ci'an and the mother of the new emperor, Cixi, who was to assume even greater control after the Tongzhi Emperor's death. The reign of the Tongzhi Emperor (1862–74) is known as a period of restoration, dominated by court officials such as Prince Gong (1833–98) and provincial leaders such as Zeng Guofan (1811–71), who had attained fame during the struggle against the Taipings. The aim of the 'restoration' was not only to rehabilitate a war-shattered economy, but also to re-establish the Confucian moral order and to strengthen China militarily vis-à-vis the West. The respite did not last long. 'Four consecutive years of natural disasters between 1876–9 brought in their wake unspeakable hardship.'³ Furthermore, the growing western presence provoked a hostile reaction that was to culminate in the Sino-French war (1884–5). The years following China's defeat in 1885 were marked by a gradual transformation of the Middle Kingdom into a semi-colony, during which there developed a popular xenophobia manifested in violent attacks on Christian missions, particularly in 1891.

Taking advantage of the crisis surrounding the Sino-Japanese war (1894–5), the western powers tightened their grip on China's economy, while a reformist current gained influence at the court. Its leaders, such as Kang Youwei (1858–1927), were invited by the Guangxu Emperor to implement reforms. This period of reform, in the summer of 1898, barely lasted 100 days before the empress-dowager Cixi brought an abrupt end to the process. At the same time, the Righteous and Harmonious Fists, better known as the Boxers, were preparing for an armed uprising against the foreign presence, an uprising that was to be crushed in 1900 by an international military expedition. The Boxers, however, were not the only ones at the beginning of the twentieth century to affirm their nationalist faith, since already on the horizon Sun Yat-sen's republican revolution was about to put an end to the imperial regime in 1911.

The Challenge of Western Medicine

As a result of the 1842–4 treaties, missionaries and foreign doctors were able to establish hospitals in the treaty ports and undertake the translation of western medical works. The most notable organisation involved in this field was the China Medical Missionary Society. Chinese doctors at this time were also introduced to western medical practice. The first Chinese to go abroad to study medicine was the Cantonese Huang Kuan (1828–79). He took a course in medicine at Edinburgh University and then, on his return to Guangzhou (Canton), practised and taught western medicine in his

home town. Others followed Huang's example, and on their return
these graduates of European and American universities became
enthusiastic advocates of western medicine, contributing thereby to
its growing influence on Chinese medicine. Hu Shenchu writes that
the propagation of western medicine undeniably 'brought new knowledge to China and benefited the development of Chinese medicine'.[4]

Let us return to the subject of the pioneers, who realised, in the
words of one of their number, Yan Fu, that they 'needed to learn
from the West'. Yan Fu himself in 1895 emphasised that 'in the
field of scholarship, one prides oneself in China on being learned in
the classics, while in the West priority is given to acquiring new
knowledge'.[5] Among the students seeking new medical knowledge
abroad was a woman, Jin Yamei (1864–1934). A native of Ningbo,
one of the first five treaty ports,[6] she acquired a medical education
from 1881 in New York. After graduating, she practised in a
hospital and contributed to a New York medical review. On
returning to China in 1888, Jin Yamei opened dispensaries in
Xiamen, Chengdu and other locations. In 1907, she worked in
Tianjin, and she died in Beijing in 1934.

The most renowned student of western medicine at the end of the
nineteenth century was Sun Zhongshan, better known as Sun Yat-
sen (1866–1925), the undisputed founder of modern China, who
said in 1924: 'If we do not learn what has been done better abroad,
we will sink into backwardness'.[7] In 1892, Sun obtained a doctorate
in medicine at the Hong Kong College of Western Medicine, having
been a student of the British doctor, James Cantlie, who would later
play a decisive role in Sun's release after he had been kidnapped in
London by Qing officials at the Chinese Embassy. Sun practised
medicine at a Macao hospital before devoting himself entirely to the
revolutionary cause.

Along with the training of 'western-style' doctors, translations of
European and Japanese medical works greatly increased in number.
Those who devoted themselves to the task of translation included
Zhao Yuanyi, who journeyed to England, France, Italy and Belgium
and adapted various European medical works into Chinese, and
Ding Fubao, who studied in Japan and was the first to introduce
Japanese medicine to China. A number of Westerners cooperated
with their Chinese counterparts in the translation of western medical
works; one other aspect of this foreign 'cooperation' was the
establishment of medical schools, first at Guangzhou (1866) and
then in other cities. At the same time, hospitals were founded at
Guangzhou, Shanghai, Beijing, Tianjin, Nanjing, Hangzhou,
Suzhou, Ningbo, Chengdu, Hankou, Fuzhou and Xiamen. Some

specialised in gynaecology, obstetrics and paediatrics (Shanghai, Tianjin, Suzhou, Chengdu), while at Chengdu a hospital for ophthalmology and otology was opened.

It might also be noted that the Taiping ban on footbinding, prostitution, alcohol, tobacco and opium was not without its positive effect on the health of those who came under the sway of the Heavenly Kingdom. With regard to medicine itself, the openness towards western medicine encouraged by Hong Ren'gan, considered a pioneer in the harmonisation of Chinese and western medicine, was put into practice by Hong Xuangjiao, none other than the sister of Hong Xiuquan. She studied western medicine at a Christian mission in Guangxi, but unfortunately it is not clear what became of her after the destruction of the Taiping Kingdom.

The 'Birth' of Traditional Chinese Medicine

Confronted with the challenge of western medicine (*xiyi*), the practice of Chinese medicine, buttressed by its age-old tradition, continued unabated in the years 1840 to 1911. Such a survival was assured by the adherents of the *Shanghanlun*, the school of 'cooling' (*hanliang pai*), the *Shen'nong Bencaojing* and other champions of traditional Chinese medicine. A physician of the time, Zhu Peiwen, author of *Huayang Zangxiang Yuezuan* (1892), in which he drew up a typology of organs according to Chinese and western concepts, wrote that each tradition had 'advantages and disadvantages'. The medical press, which made its appearance at the end of the eighteenth century with *Wuyi Huijiang*, contributed to the defence of traditional Chinese medicine, in particular the Shanghai *Journal of Medicine* (*Yixue Bao*, later *Yixue Gongbao*) whose first issue was published in June 1904. In 1908, the *Medical Review of Shanghai* was inaugurated and, in Shaoxing, the *Sansan Yibao*.

Western trends in medicine did not in any way deter those who continued, like their predecessors in previous centuries, to draw inspiration from the *Shanghanlun* (*On Cold-induced Illnesses*). They included Zhou Xuehai, who published *Shanghan Buli* at the turn of the twentieth century, Lu Maoxiu (1818–86), who published his research on the *Shanghanlun* in 1884, and Chen Gongpu, author of *Shanghanlun Zhangju* in 1851.

The school of 'cooling', whose evolution from Liu Wansu in the twelfth century to Yu Lin at the end of the eighteenth was described earlier (Yu Lin's *Yizhen Yide*, moreover, was reissued in 1828 and 1879), was eminently represented in the nineteenth century by Wang Mengying, also known as Wang Shixiong (1808–66). Wang devoted an entire work to fever-related illnesses, the *Wenre Jingwei*.

Completed and published in 1852, *Wenre Jingwei*, which exists in
several editions, exerted a lasting influence. Two other works
connected with this school deserve mention: *Wenre Fengyuan* (*The
Source of Fevers*) by Liu Baoyi (1842–1901), and *Shibinglun*
(*Seasonal Illnesses*), written by Lei Feng in 1882. Lei Feng
expounded on a theme dear to traditional Chinese medicine since
the *Huangdi Neijing*, the need to live in harmony with the influences
of the four seasons. Thus, in summer:

> Man goes to bed at night and rises at dawn.
> One should avoid the sun . . .
> One must assist in the flow of influences,
> which, it appears, are best kept external (to oneself).
> This is the proper way to accord with the influences
> of summer . . .
> He who acts contrary to these influences will bring
> harm to his heart;
> And, in autumn, will cause intermittent fever . . .[8]

Lei Feng devoted a chapter in *Shibinglun* to intermittent fevers
(jienüe), distinguishing 'summer malaria' (*shunue*) from 'cold
malaria' (*han'nue*), or 'female malaria' (*pin'nüe*), because its
symptom was an excessive shivering with cold, equated with *yin*.
At the end of each chapter in Lei Feng's treatise on 'seasonal'
illnesses, various remedies are prescribed.

The *Illustrated Account of Flora* (*Zhiwu Mingshi Tukao*) of Wu
Qijun (1789–1846), with its description of the therapeutic qualities
of the various plants presented, belongs to the tradition initiated by
the *Classic of Herbal Medicine*. Moreover, throughout the nineteenth
century, earlier medical works of this tradition were reissued in new
editions, works that included Li Shizhen's *Bencao Gangmu*, Wang
An's *Bencao Beiyao*, Wu Yiluo's *Bencao Congxin* and Zhao
Xuemin's *Bencao Gangmu Shiyi*. Phytotherapy, in fact, remained
the basis of Chinese medicine. It was the desire to revive this plant-
based medicine that inspired a physician like Fei Boxiong, for
whom emulation of traditional methods did not in any way mean an
unquestioning and wholesale endorsement. Thus, in his *Yichun
Shengyi* (1863), he advised against the inconsiderate use of the
following medicinal plants: *Cimicifuga foetida, Bupleurum chinese,
Anemarrhena asphodeloides, Phellodendron amurense, Aconitum
carmichaeli, Cinnamomum cassia* and gypsum, the use of which
had been rediscovered by Yu Lin in the eighteenth century.

For his part, Wu Shangxian or Wu Shiji (1806–86) championed
external therapy, presenting his ideas in a book published in 1870

entitled *Liyue Pianwen*. Wu referred to the use of liniments, ointments, fumigation, thermal baths, massage and various medical concoctions, all of which he had probably tested in the pharmacy which he opened in 1865 at Yangzhou. This was not the only dispensary; the most renowned of the time was located in the capital, the *Tongren tang*, which catered especially to the imperial family.

Techniques for Prolonging Life and Superstition

The search for longevity was still a preoccupation of Daoists at the beginning of the twentieth century. Although *Weisheng Shenglixue Mingzhi* (*A Clear Explanation of Physiology and Hygiene*) by Zhao Bichen (b. 1860) is not, despite its title, a medical work, the existence of such a work describing Daoist practices aimed at 'safeguarding life' (*weisheng*) and hence acquiring longevity cannot be ignored. Although the physiological descriptions presented by Zhao Bichen and followers of the Daoist school of internal alchemy (*neidan*) may strike contemporaries by their inaccuracy, Catherine Despeux notes that 'it is quite probable that Zhao and others knew how to affect the working of the endocrine glands and that their awareness of various physiological processes was superior to that of the ordinary person'.[9]

Another method to prolong life that became popular at this time was *Taijiquan* (Chinese shadow-boxing). Although *taijiquan* has become a fitness exercise in the People's Republic, it should not be forgotten that originally the exercise was a combat skill, some of the movements of which are not unconnected with those of *daoyin* and even certain practices to improve internal organs. 'Various mental processes are used', writes Catherine Despeux, 'in order to produce the desired physiological effects'.[10]

In his *Manuel des Superstitions Chinoises* (1926), the Jesuit Henri Doré observed that 'illness causes man to become incredulous'. In a chapter devoted to illnesses, Doré referred to the curious practice of using human flesh in decoctions. 'This remedy was regarded as the most efficacious, capable of curing the most helpless cases. The patient, however, had to be kept ignorant of the remedy's origin; if not, the potion would lose all its potency.'[11] People also consulted fortune-telling almanacs, and there was doubtless a profitable trade in charms and talismans. Finally, processions were often organised whenever an epidemic raged.

Notes

1. Victor Hugo, *OEuvres complètes* (Paris: Le Club Français du Livre, 1969), 12:851–2.
2. Jean Chesneaux, Marianne Bastid and Marie-Claire Bergère, *China from the Opium Wars to the 1911 Revolution* (Hassocks, Sussex: Harvester, 1977), p 89.
3. Ibid., pp 165–6.
4. Yu Shenchu, *Zhongguo Yixue Jianshi*, op. cit., p 362.
5. Yan Fu, the son and grandson of physicians, had been sent to England for naval training.
6. Catherine Gipoulon, *Qiu Jin: Femme et Révolutionnaire en Chine au Dix-neuvième Siècle* (Paris: Editions des Femmes, 1976), p 229, notes that 'it was in 1844 at Ningbo that the first Chinese school for girls was opened by an English missionary'. She adds that the missionary schools between 1890 and 1905 'trained the first generation of Chinese women to become physicians and teachers in hospitals and mission schools'.
7. Sun Yat-sen, *The Three People's Principles* (Taipei: China Publishing Company), p 48.
8. Claude Larre and Elisabeth Rochat de La Vallée, *Assaisonner les Esprits*, op. cit., p 24.
9. Zhao Bichen, *Traité d'Alchimie et de Physiologie Taoiste*, translated and introduced by Catherine Despeux (Paris: Les Deux Océans, 1979), p 83.
10. Catherine Despeux, *T'ai-k'ï k'iuan, Technique de Longue Vie, Technique de Combat* (Paris: Institut des hautes études chinoises, 1975), p 49.
11. H. Doré, *Manuel des Superstitions Chinoises*, op. cit., p 41.

— 11 —

From the 1911 Revolution to the Establishment of The People's Republic, 1911–49

From One Republic to Another

The Republic of China was officially inaugurated on 1 January 1912 in the wake of the 1911 Revolution, with Sun Yat-sen as its first president. In March 1912, however, Sun ceded the presidency to Yuan Shikai. Yuan's death in 1916 opened the way for warlord rule, when provincial militarists held sway. The Treaty of Versailles following the First World War allowed Japan to take over German concessions in China, and it was in this context that large-scale student demonstrations broke out on 4 May 1919, followed by workers' strikes and an anti-Japanese boycott. The May Fourth Movement, according to Jean Chesneaux, 'started a whole series of new processes, whose importance was to prove decisive for the whole course of Chinese history up to and even beyond 1949'.[1] It was in the wake of the May Fourth Movement that the Chinese Communist Party was founded, its first congress taking place in 1921 at Shanghai.

From the establishment of the Nationalist government in 1927 to the communist victory in 1949, China experienced a long period of instability. The Jiangxi Soviet (1927–34), under Mao Zedong's leadership, had to confront the encirclement campaigns launched against it by Jiang Jieshi (Chiang Kai-shek). Such campaigns forced the communists to evacuate the Jiangxi Soviet and embark on the tortuous Long March (1934–5), which eventually brought them to Yan'an in the north-west. Meanwhile, Japan's invasion of Manchuria in 1931 was to culminate in an eight-year war, beginning in 1937 with Japan's full-scale onslaught on China. After Japan's surrender, civil war broke out between nationalists and communists as each side bid for sole power. The Chinese People's Republic was officially inaugurated on 1 October 1949.

Furore over China's Medical Heritage

'If we wish to learn from the West's positive features, we must grasp the initiative and not remain backward',[2] declared Sun Yat-sen in 1924. Due to his own 'western-style' medical training, Sun was probably thinking of medicine as an example. Whatever the case, Chinese authorities between 1912 and 1926 did in fact take initiatives to improve public hygiene, especially in urban areas such as Shanghai, Tianjin, Qingdao, Guangzhou, Hankou, Beijing, Changchun and Kunming, where running water was gradually introduced. The cleansing of streets was encouraged. In 1919, a central bureau to combat epidemics was created, while the Ministry of Education issued regulations on medical instruction. Public and private schools of medicine were established. At the same time, centres of health care and training were opened by western and Japanese doctors. Doctors' associations were formed and medical journals published, such as the *China Medical Review* (*Zhonghua Yixue Zazhi*), founded in 1915 by former graduates of medicine from American and European universities.

Rural China, however, hardly benefited from the western-inspired changes in medicine taking place in the first quarter of the twentieth century. Clearly, the old doctor referred to by Jan Myrdal was not trained in one of the medical schools being opened in the large urban centres, but rather in the time-honoured ways of tradition:

> When I was twenty-three or twenty-four, I had gone to the doctor with a stomach complaint. He treated me for two years, and I began to get interested in medicine . . . To begin with, I was just his pupil and watched while he treated his patients. He explained to me what he was doing and let me feel the pulse and understand about it. Then, gradually, I was allowed to treat the less serious cases myself, under his supervision.[3]

This doctor, who had been trained on the job, was unaware, no doubt like the rest of his rural contemporaries, that from the first years of the Republic, the Minister of Education, Wang Daxie, had urged the abandonment of traditional Chinese medicine. Such a call had aroused fierce protest. Nevertheless, this policy was pursued by the Nationalist government, which in 1929 adopted a series of hostile measures strictly controlling the practice of traditional Chinese medicine. The opening of schools for traditional medicine was prohibited, while censorship was to prevent the diffusion of medical information deemed 'unscientific'. In response to such measures, angry supporters of traditional medicine in March 1929 sent delegates from 132 associations to meet in Shanghai. This assembly formed the National Union of Associations for Chinese Medicine and decreed that henceforth 17 March would be celebrated as the 'birthday of national medicine'. A delegation went to the capital, Nanjing, to request the suspension of the restrictive measures. Such protests were in vain, since the government definitively prohibited those physicians practising traditional medicine from making use of western medicine or instruments. Moreover, they were forbidden from establishing medical schools or opening hospitals. Other restrictions followed.

This attempt, however, to eliminate traditional Chinese medicine failed. Wang Pei, in a 1983 treatise published by the World Health Organisation, discerned three reasons for this failure:

> First, the population of the vast rural hinterland, as well as the elites and ordinary people of countless towns, continued to believe unwaveringly in traditional medicine. Second, the use of Chinese traditional medicine and medicinal plants produced satisfactory enough results in the treatment of illnesses, particularly those which modern medicine apparently could not cure. Traditional medicine could alleviate the symptoms and even bring about improvement. Moreover, medicinal plants were widely available, relatively inexpensive, practical and easy to use, and had few adverse affects. Consequently, their use remained popular for a large majority of the population. Third, traditional Chinese medicine was based on a unique theoretical system, notably with regard to the concepts of *yin* and *yang*, of vital energy and of blood that modern medicine could neither replace nor explain. It therefore survived, despite the persecution to which it was subject before the liberation.[4]

Another reason for the survival of traditional medicine would be the resistance carried out by its practitioners and its associations, such as the Shanghai review, *Yijie chunqiu* (*Spring and Autumn of the Medical World*). First appearing in 1926, the review was the principal voice of opposition to the government's restrictive measures, especially in 1929.

New Developments in Traditional Chinese Medicine

The challenge posed by the influx of western medicine in China led many physicians, without abandoning their national heritage, to propose rejecting the shortcomings of traditional Chinese medicine while assimilating the beneficial aspects of western medicine. This current of thought was known as the *Zhongxi huitong pai*, or School (*pai*) of Sino-Western (*zhongxi*) Convergence (*hui*) and Intercourse (*tong*).

Tang Zonghai (1846-97)[5] is considered the pioneer of this outlook. A native of Sichuan province, Tang studied both Chinese and western medicine. In 1884, he wrote a treatise on blood disorders (*Xuezhenglun*) and then, in 1892, he published the *Zhongxi Huitong Yijing Jingyi* in which he called for 'convergence' and 'intercourse', that is the reconciliation of the two traditions, each with their shortcomings to abandon and advantages to conserve, to form one system. He justified such a system by referring to the necessity of 'calculating the advantages of the ancient and new' (*sunyi he gujiu*) and of 'weighing up the pros and cons of what is Chinese and foreign' (*canzhou he zhongwai*). These ideas were shared by Zhang Xichun (1860-1933), who elaborated on them in his *Yixue Zhongzhong Canxi Lu*. Zhang, who valued tradition without ever being in its thrall, was a passionate supporter of Sino-Western medical exchange. His book outlined the various clinical applications of such an exchange that he himself practised on his patients.

This school of thought gained the support of the scholar and political activist, Zhang Binglin, known also as Zhang Taiyan. Born in 1869, Zhang Binglin became acquainted in 1899 with Sun Yat-sen while on a trip to Japan. He joined Sun's organisation, the *Tongmenghui* (Alliance League), in 1906 and wrote for its organ, *Minbao* (*People's Journal*). Zhang, who died in 1936, was a controversial thinker. The celebrated writer Lu Xun, in a text published on 9 October 1936, reproached him for 'at first behaving like a revolutionary' but then 'regressing to become no more than a quiescent scholar'.[6] Whatever the case, and even if one agrees with Lu Xun that 'Zhang Binglin's contribution is more significant in the history of the revolution than in that of learning', Zhang defended the outlook of people like Tang Zonghai, whom he proclaimed as the enlightened champion of Chinese medicine willing to accept western scientific theory.

A final representative of the 'convergence and intercourse school' deserves mention, Wu Ruifu (1871-1951). Wu was the author of several 'comparative' medical works on such aspects as pulsing (*Zhongxi Maixue Jiangyi*), internal medicine (*Zhongxi Neikexue*) and brain and spinal disorders (*Naosuibinglun*). His last years were spent in Singapore, where he founded a medical research institute that published innumerable works under his supervision.

The reform of traditional Chinese medicine was thus initiated. Was this not the best means of preserving it? Figures such as Yun Tieqiao (1878-1935) and Yang Zemin (1893-1948) were convinced that it was. Yun Tieqiao, translator of English novels and promoter of literary reviews, became interested in medicine at the age of forty when his eldest son died. The *Shanghanlun* attracted his interest at first, and he published several works on this fundamental medical text. In 1925, he launched a highly successful correspondence school for Chinese medicine in Shanghai. Yun's numerous publications, with such revealing titles as *Shengli Xinshu* (*New Work on Physiology*), *Huolan Xinshu* (*New Work on Cholera*) and *Maixue Fawei* (*Disclosures on Pulsing*), testified to his concern that the Chinese medical tradition be reformed.

Yang Zemin, who came to medicine much sooner that Yun Tieqiao, was equally an innovator. He became well-known in the world of Chinese traditional medicine and taught at the Zhejiang Specialist School of Chinese Medicine (*Zhejiang zhongyi zhuanmen xuexiao*). Towards the end of his life, Yang supported the reconciliation of Chinese and western medicine:

> Chinese medicine attaches importance to the discovery of symptoms, while western medicine distinguishes among illnesses. The aim of discovering symptoms is to treat the illness with the appropriate drug, that of distinguishing among illnesses is to localise the source of the illness.

According to Yang, both approaches had their advantages and disadvantages, and he concluded that the ideal solution was to combine the strong points of each.

The teaching of traditional Chinese medicine benefited from the competitive activities of enthusiasts such as Fu Lanyuan, Ding Ganren, Zhang Shanlei and Xie Liheng. Fu Lanyuan (1861–1931) was active in Hangzhou, where he founded in 1916 the Zhejiang Specialist School of Chinese Medicine. Anxious to train a highly-qualified medical personnel, Fu insisted on the need for both theoretical and practical instruction. He was also concerned with medical ethics. Ding Ganren (1866–1926), a specialist in scarlet fever, about which he wrote an entire work, *Housha Zhengzhi Gaiyao* (*Fundamental Ideas on How to Diagnose and Treat Scarlet Fever*), also distinguished himself as a teacher. He opened a school of Chinese medicine in Shanghai as well as a women's medical school. In 1919, Zhang Shanlei (1872–1934) was invited to take charge of the Lanxi Special School of Chinese Medicine (*Lanxi zhongyi zhuanmen xuexiao*) that Ge Shaoqing had just opened. Author of a number of medical works, notably *Yangke Gangyao* (*A Concise Study of Dermatology*), Zhang's total commitment has become renowned: Yu Shenchu notes that 'during the day he kept busy giving consultations and teaching; at night he wrote by the light of a wood fire'.[7] Xie Liheng (1880–1953) also contributed to the development and, from 1929, the defence of instruction in Chinese traditional medicine. First invited to Shanghai in 1917 by Ding Ganren, he was then hired by the Shenzhou Medical Association, which had founded a university for Chinese medicine. He afterwards participated in the protest movement against the government measures restricting the practice of traditional medicine. Xie also supervised the publication of *Zhongguo Yixue Dacidian* (*Encyclopaedia of Chinese Medicine*).

Besides the people just mentioned, the world of traditional Chinese medicine during the first half of the twentieth century witnessed the emergence of other significant personalities. He Lianchen (1861–1929), who was president of the Shaoxing Medical Society and editor-in-chief of the *Shaoxing Yiyao Xuebao* (*Shaoxing Journal of Medicine and Pharmacy*, 1908–23), exerted a considerable influence on the school associated with the *Shanghanlun* in his native town of Shaoxing. He's colleague from Shanghai, Cao Yingfu (1866–1937), was an enthusiastic follower of 'classical remedies' (*jingfang*), which he contrasted with 'contemporary remedies' (*shifang*). Cao also bequeathed to posterity a copious record of his clinical experiences, the *Jingfang Shiyanlu* (*Experiments with Classical Remedies*). Qiu Jisheng (1873–1947), founder of the March Third Medical Association (*Sansan yishe*) and of the *March Third Medical Journal* (*Sansan Yibao*, 1923–9), was not attached to any particular school. Moreover, he was convinced of the utility of Sino-Western medical exchanges. Bao Shisheng (1874–1934) was an expert on the *Shanghanlun*. He gave courses on Zhang Zhongjing's medical classic at the Shenzhou Specialist School of Chinese Medicine and devoted much of his publishing career to it. Chen Wujiu (1880–1947), for his part, preferred to concentrate on the theories of Hejian (Liu Wansu) and Danxi (Zhu Zhenheng). Finally, there was Zhang Boxi (1880–1949), who helped found in 1926 the review *Shijie Chunqiu* (*Spring and Autumn of the Medical World*). Zhang championed the cause of traditional Chinese medicine until 1937, when he disappeared from public view.

Herbal Medicine at a Time of Scientific Research

It was only during the 1920s, under the influence of graduates of European, American and Japanese universities, that pharmaceutical research became more systematic and produced its first significant results.[8] In 1923, Chen Kehui, C. F. Schmidt and B. E. Read (author of numerous works on Chinese herbal medicine) began a study of the Chinese angelica (*Angelica sinensis*) and the ephedra (*Ephedra sinica*). Chen and Schmidt ultimately carried out pharmaceutical research on ephedrine, work that was acknowledged by specialists throughout the world. Research was also carried out on aconite (*Aconitum carmichaeli*) and on other plants used in traditional Chinese medicine, particularly a plant of the poppy family known at least since the Song dynasty (as described in the *Kaibao Bencao*) as the *yanhusuo* or *yuanhu* (*corydalis*).[9]

The name of Zhao Cheng'gu is associated with research done on the *yanhusuo*, as well as on the fritillary, an alkaloid extract from the bulb of a liliaceous plant, the *beimu* (*fritillaria*). During the 1930s and 1940s, the Central Research Institute (*Zhongyang yanjiuyuan*), the Beiping Research Institute (*Beiping yanjiuyuan*) and the Central Laboratory of Hygiene (*Zhongyang weisheng shiyanchu*) focused on the therapeutic quality of plants such as *Ligusticum chuanxiong, Codonopsis pilosula, Rehmannia glutinosa, Pinellia ternata, Plantago asiatica* and, in particular, *Dichroa febrifuga*, a shrub of the saxifrage family, whose root has long been used to combat malaria.[10] Chemical and clinical research, pharmacognosy, pharmacology and parasitology have all demonstrated the positive role of this plant in the treatment of malaria.[11]

These research activities were accompanied by a variety of publications on traditional and modern medicine. One of the most important was the *Zhongguo Yaoxue Dacidian* (*Chinese Pharmaceutical Encyclopaedia*), published by Chen Cunren in the early 1930s. Yu Shenchu lists more than seventy journals on traditional Chinese medicine and nearly fifty on western medicine that were published between 1908 and 1947.[12] Most of them had a brief existence, and only a few lasted more than twenty years.

The *Shijie Chunqiu* (*Spring and Autumn of the Medical World*), a monthly journal of traditional Chinese medicine, was founded in 1926 and saw its last issue in 1937, as indeed did many other journals because of the Sino-Japanese war. This was the case especially with the *Zhongyi Shijie* (*The World of Chinese Medicine*), the *Shenzhou Guoyi Xuebao* (*Shenzhou Review of National Medicine*), the *Xiandai Yiyao* (*Contemporary Pharmacy and Medicine*), the *Zhenjiu Zazhi* (*Review of Acupuncture and Moxibustion*) and those dealing with western medicine such as the *Beiping Yikan* (*Beiping Medical Journal*) and the *Yishi Gonglun* (*Medical Public Opinion*), organ of the Association for Medical Progress in China (*Zhongguo yishi gaijinhui*).

The history of medicine not only found a niche in the medical journals but also attracted the interest of specialists, of whom the most celebrated was Wang Jimin (Wang Jiaxiang). In the early 1930s, Wang, together with Wu Liande, published *The History of*

Chinese Medicine (in English). Wang Jimin is also associated with the foundation, in 1936, of the Study Society for the History of Medicine in China (*Zhonghua yishi xuehui*) and, in 1938, with the creation in Shanghai of a museum of medical history. Moreover, Wang helped inaugurate, with Li Tao, the *Yishi Zazhi* (*Review of Medical History*) in 1947.

Under the Protection of the Red Army

Edgar Snow, in his celebrated book *Red Star over China* (New York, 1938), wrote concerning Mao Zedong:

> There would never be any one 'saviour' in China, yet undeniably one felt a certain force of destiny in Mao. It was nothing quick or flashy, but a kind of solid elemental vitality. One felt that whatever there was extraordinary in this man grew out of the uncanny degree to which he synthesized and expressed the urgent demands of millions of Chinese, and especially the peasantry.[13]

It was Mao Zedong himself who observed in 1934 that in order to defeat the enemy, it was necessary to do more than simply 'mobilise the people for war'; in particular, one had to 'solve the problems facing the masses – food, shelter, and clothing . . .', as well as problems of 'sickness and hygiene, and marriage'. He added later on in the same article: 'Many people suffer from boils and other ailments. What are we going to do about it?'[14]

The resolution of this problem was already a priority several years earlier, soon after the creation of the Red Army and the opening of its first hospital in the Jing'gang mountains in October 1927. Poor sanitary conditions among the population in areas controlled by the communists soon became evident. Dispensaries and hospitals were opened. The government of the Jiangxi Soviet Republic established an Administrative Office for the Promotion of Hygiene (*Weisheng quanliju*) in 1931, and its recommendations were publicised in various propaganda organs such as *Hongse Weisheng* (*Red Hygiene*) and *Jiankangbao* (*Health Journal*). After the Long March, the Red Army established its headquarters in 1935 at Yanan, where a central hospital was opened. At the same time, health centres were created in each district. As for the combatants themselves, one of the rules for discipline imposed on them concerned hygiene: 'Be sanitary, and, especially, establish latrines a safe distance from people's houses'.[15]

One of the players in the medical drama taking place in revolutionary China at the end of the 1930s was the celebrated Canadian doctor, Norman Bethune (1890–1939). After Bethune's

death, Mao Zedong was to praise his 'total selflessness' and his
'utter devotion to others', encouraging all communists to 'learn from
his example'.[16] Bethune, who won fame during the Spanish Civil
War when he carried out blood transfusions on the front line,
arrived in Yanan during the spring of 1938. He met Mao Zedong,
who suggested he organise mobile medical units. In this way,
Bethune became a doctor for the celebrated Eighth Route Army. In
a report drawn up during a tour of inspection, Bethune bore witness
to the sanitary conditions of the wounded:

> The wounded are crawling with lice. They all have only one
> uniform, and that they have on. It is filthy with the accumulated
> dirt of nine months' fighting. Their bandages have been washed
> so often that they are now nothing but dirty rags. Three men,
> one with the loss of both feet through frost-bite gangrene, have
> no clothes at all to wear. There is only a coverlet for them.
> Their food is boiled millet – that's all. All are anaemic and
> underfed. Most of them are slowly dying of sepsis and
> starvation. Many have tuberculosis.[17]

In June 1938, Bethune made his way to the Shanxi-Chahar-Hebei
region, where he worked in difficult conditions.

> There were no anaesthetics, apart from what he had brought,
> no regular operating rooms, none of the regular instruments
> required for surgery. Bandages were washed after use, hung
> out to dry, then used again. There was only home-made thread
> for stitching up wounds. Medical supplies consisted mostly of
> pills of local manufacture and dubious value. Probes were
> made with wire. For tweezers and pincers pieces of iron were
> used. There were no training facilities for doctors or medical
> attendants of any kind.[18]

Appointed medical adviser for the military region of Shanxi-Chahar-
Hebei, Bethune created a model hospital with an operating room
and established a training school for medical personnel. His mobile
medical unit then departed for the front. On 8 December 1938,
Bethune noted in his journal: 'Despite the fact that there were no
secondary dressing stations between our unit and the Base Hospital,
one-third of the wounded arrived at the hospital without any trace
of infection! That is something new here. It is a great advance, but
we can do even better.'[19]

Bethune died of blood poisoning on 13 November 1939. The
Indian doctor, Kotnis, another participant in the international
medical aid to China, took Bethune's place, dying in 1942.

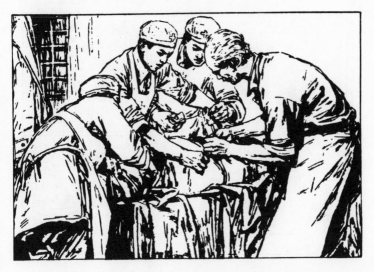

FIGURE 11.1   Norman Bethune performs an operation. From
Norman Bethune in China (Beijing: Foreign Languages Press,
1975).

A Dismal Balance-sheet on Health

Saint-John Perse wrote in a letter to his mother dated 9 April 1918:

> I very much hope that you will not worry too much about the
> plague epidemic that has been raging in north China for the
> last few months ... It is particularly severe in the western
> provinces and in the suburbs of Beijing, but there have still
> only been a few cases within Beijing itself ... In fact, this
> consumptive plague, although the most serious, is also the
> easiest to avoid individually. The simple wearing of a mask is
> enough to protect oneself in the home. Real danger confronts
> only the heaving mass of poor trudging the roads.[20]

The testimony of this French diplomat and poet invites the drawing-
up of a balance-sheet on China's health situation during the first
half of the twentieth century. Such a balance-sheet appears to be
grim: cholera, plague, smallpox, black fever, bilharzia and
tuberculosis are its most serious features.

From the start of the resistance war against Japan (1937) to
1949, cholera caused more than 100,000 deaths. In 1938, 2,400
died of it in Shanghai alone. Plague, which affected the north-east

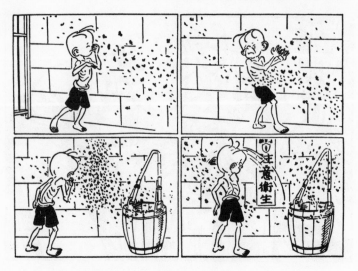

FIGURE 11.2   So much for hygiene. Sanmao, the well-known
creation of the cartoonist Zhang Leping, 'sees through' a poster of
Chiang Kai-shek's New Life Movement carrying these words: 'Pay
attention to hygiene'. From *Sanmao Liulangji Xuanji* (Shanghai:
Shaonian Ertong Chubanshe, 1978).

on several occasions, caused nearly 100,000 deaths during just the
three years of 1910, 1920 and 1947. In Harbin, during the winter of
1910, more than 6,000 inhabitants out of a population of 20,000
died of the plague. Smallpox affected every region. Between 1939
and 1949, 380,000 contracted the disease throughout the country.
The number afflicted with black fever (Kala-azar) in 1949 has been
estimated at 530,000. According to an investigation carried out in
324 districts in the provinces of Jiangsu, Jiangxi and Zhejiang,
10,000,000 people were suffering from bilharzia on the eve of the
establishment of the People's Republic. At the same time, typhoid,
diphtheria, scarlet fever and malaria raged throughout China. The
same applied to tuberculosis, which killed approximately 1,000,000
men and women every year between 1915 and 1925.[21]

An illustration of the constant danger of tuberculosis is to be
found in the following extract from Ba Jin's novel, *Winter Night*:

He spat, regained his breath and drank. Then, gasping for
breath, he cried out: 'I'm going to die.' 'What are you saying,'
said Shousheng tenderly, 'you have nothing to fear. In two
days you will be better.' 'I'm not afraid,' he said, shaking his
head, 'but I know that I will never be cured. I've a horrible taste
in my mouth and I'm starting to spit blood again.'

Instinctively, Shousheng glanced in the direction of the spittoon. She shuddered but continued to make an effort to console Shuenn: 'Whether you're spitting blood or not doesn't matter. The last time this happened you took some prescriptions and everything was better, wasn't it?' Shuenn looked at his wife with affection. 'Even you don't believe in Chinese medicine. Do you really think my illness can be cured by gulping down a few insignificant medicines?'

The mother remained silent, lowering her head and wiping her tears. The silence compelled Shousheng to persist with her optimistic words: 'Okay, so it's tuberculosis, but it's curable.' A sad smile appeared on Shuenn's face and his eyes grew dim: 'Curable? It's a curse that poor people like us catch this costly disease. How can you say I'm going to be cured? . . .'[22]

The hapless Shuenn knew that, unlike Lao Tongbao, the hero of Mao Dun's short story *Spring Silkworms*, he could not rely on his own strength 'to fight off the spectre of illness'.[23]

Notes

1. Marianne Bastid, Marie-Claire Bergère and Jean Chesneaux, *China from the 1911 Revolution to Liberation* (Hassocks, Sussex: Harvester, 1977), p 74. In a letter dated 3 January 1917, Saint-John Perse wrote: 'The thought of Marx and Engels already holds a secret attraction for Chinese intellectual youth. In the long term, via numerous setbacks and transitional interludes, and perhaps even before the achievement of national unity, nothing will halt the final march of the Chinese community towards a collectivism akin to orthodox Leninism.' Saint-John Perse, *Œuvres Complètes* (Paris: Bibliothèque de la Pléiade), p 810.
2. Sun Yat-sen, *The Three People's Principles*, op. cit., p 49.
3. Jan Myrdal, *Report from a Chinese Village* (New York, 1965), pp 287, 288.
4. Wang Pei, 'Médecine chinoise traditionnelle', in *Médecine Traditionnelle et Couverture des Soins de Santé* (World Health Organisation, 1983), p 71.
5. Chen Xianfu, 'Tang Zonghai shengzu xinkao', *Zhonghua Yishi Zazhi*, no 1 (1987), pp 18–20. Various dates have been given for Tang Zonghai. The author of this article maintains that he was born in 1846 and died in 1897.
6. Lu Xun, *Pamphlets et Libelles (1925–1936)*, introduced and translated by Michelle Loi (Paris: François Maspero, 1977), p 219. An article devoted to Zhang Binglin in *Zhongguo Jindai Zhuming Zhexuejia Pingzhuan* (Critical Biographies of Famous Philosophers of Modern China) (Jinan: Qilu Shushe Chubanshe, 1983) argues that 'in the final analysis he abandoned a materialist outlook and turned to idealism' (pp 48–9).
7. Yu Shenchu, *Zhongguo Yixue Jianshi*, op. cit., p 427.
8. See Chen Xinqian, 'Benshiji 20–40 niandai guoren dui zhong yaode yanjiu' (Research on Chinese materia medica between

1920 and 1940), *Zhonghua Yishi Zazhi*, no 2 (1987), pp 107–13.

9. Work done on the rhizome of the *Corydalis yanhusuo* has resulted in isolation of more than ten alkaloids, including protopine, corydaline and ±tetrahydropalmatine. ±Tetrahydropalmatine, which has an analgesic effect on spasmodic pains, is commercially produced today. Research has also demonstrated the beneficial effect of dihydrocorydaline on the cardiovascular system. See Jiang Xierong, *Acta Pharmacologica Sinica*, 17 (1), 1982, pp 61–5.

10. As described by Loureiro in his *Flora Cochinchinensis* (1790).

11. In his *Flora Cochinchinensis*, the botanist Loureiro mentions the use of *Dichroa febrifuga* to treat malaria. The active elements of the root of the *Dichroa febrifuga* were not extensively researched in various countries until 1948. Febrifugine (the alkaloid derivative of quinazoline) is considerably more active than quinine but cannot be used because of its high toxicity and insufficient quantity. The alkaloids derived from the *Dichroa febrifuga* have been used to make synthetic substances. Apart from febrifugine, a derivative of the plant with anti-arrhythmic properties has been prepared through partial synthesis. See Xiao Peigen, 'Recent Developments on Medicinal Plants in China', *Journal of Ethnopharmacology*, 7 (1983), pp 95–109.

12. Yu Shenchu, *Zhongguo Yixue Jianshi*, op. cit., pp 401–8.

13. Edgar Snow, *Red Star over China* (New York: Random House, 1968), p 90.

14. Mao Zedong, 'Be Concerned with the Well-being of the Masses, Pay Attention to Methods of Work' (27 January 1934), *Selected Readings from the Works of Mao Tse-Tung* (Peking: Foreign Language Press, 1971), pp 52, 53.

15. Edgar Snow, *Red Star over China*, op. cit., p 173.

16. Mao Zedong, 'In Memory of Norman Bethune' (21 December 1939), *Selected Readings from the Works of Mao Tse-Tung*, pp 179–81.

17. Sydney Gordon and Ted Allan, *The Scalpel, The Sword* (London, 1954), p 159.

18. Ibid., p 164.

19. Ibid., p 215.

20. Saint-John Perse, *OEuvres Complètes*, op. cit., pp 856–7.

21. From *Zhongguo Yixueshi*, op. cit., pp 134–5.

22. Ba Jin, *Nuit Glacée* (*Winter Night*), translated from the Chinese by M.-J. Lalitte (Paris: Gallimard, 1978), pp 174–5.

23. Mao Dun, *Spring Silkworms and Other Stories* (Peking: Foreign Languages Press, 1979).

12

Mao Zedong's China

The Communist Party in Power

Jacques Guillermaz notes that an immense task awaited the Communist Party when it came to power'.[1] With national unity re-established, the priority was to rehabilitate the economy. It was with this aim in mind that Mao Zedong himself, on 6 June 1950, laid down the conditions for a radical improvement in the economic situation, which included agrarian reform.[2] Rather than going into details on the political, economic, social and cultural changes in China since 1949, only the broad outlines will be sketched.

Until 1955, as Gilbert Etienne has observed, 'the regime sought to implement a gradual transition towards socialism',[3] but on 31 July 1955 Mao accelerated the process, declaring that 'an upsurge in the new, socialist mass movement is imminent throughout the countryside'.[4] In 1957, he launched the 'Hundred Flowers' campaign followed by, in 1958, the Great Leap Forward and the People's Communes. By 1964–5, the economy had recovered from the excesses of the Great Leap and had attained a certain equilibrium. In China at the time, Edgar Snow remarked that 'the "hardship years" of 1959–1962 were past, food was relatively plentiful, and consumer essentials and services were more widely available'.[5]

It was at this point that the Cultural Revolution (1966–9) erupted. While Maria-Antonietta Macciocchi in 1971 saw in this 'second Chinese revolution' (in the words of K. S. Karol[6]) 'evidence of a significant choice being made in the path of Chinese socialism',[7] S. Leys regarded it as a 'struggle for power'.[8] The anti-Lin Biao, anti-Confucius campaign of 1974 indicated that it had not yet ended, and in 1975 the novelist Han Suyin could write that 'just as in 1949, there is in China today a right[ist] tendency which wants no change'.[9] The year 1976 witnessed the deaths of Zhou Enlai and

Mao Zedong, soon followed by the removal of the Gang of Four
from power. China thereupon entered a new era.

Demography and Family Planning

The exact population of China has long posed problems. The 1953
census gave a total of nearly 600 million, but Jacques Guillermaz,
writing in 1972, observed that 'since 1958 no general or partial
statistics have been given on birth, mortality or marriage rates'.
Guillermaz concluded that 'it looks as though the Chinese leaders
no longer dare to face the agonizing problem of multitude'.[10] The
1982 census finally put an end to unofficial calculations; the
population totalled more than one billion.

On 9 October 1957, at a Central Committee meeting, Mao gave
his thoughts on the question of birth control and proposed a ten-
year plan:

> However, it should not be promoted in the minority nationality
> areas or in sparsely populated regions. Even in densely
> populated regions it is necessary to try it out in selected places
> and then spread it step by step until family planning gradually
> becomes universal. Family planning requires open education,
> which simply means airing views freely and holding great
> debates. As far as procreation is concerned, the human race
> has been in a state of total anarchy and failed to exercise
> control. The complete realization of family planning in the
> future will be out of the question without the weight of society
> as a whole behind it, that is, without general consent and joint
> effort.[11]

A few days later, on 13 October 1957, Mao returned to the
question of family planning: 'The prospects for the success of family
planning are good. There should be a great debate on this matter
too, and there should be periods of trial, expansion and
popularization, each lasting several years.'[12] Modern contraceptive
methods were introduced. Edgar Snow reported that

> A nation-wide campaign spread knowledge of modern 'family
> planning' methods to every village and town. Graphic posters,
> picture books, movies and demonstration lectures carried the
> methods right into the peasant's home. After a trial period
> these efforts waned at a time which coincided with the
> development of commune plans.[13]

Moreover, the campaign for birth control was met with indifference,
a 'serene inertia' in the words of Alain Peyrefitte,[14] and even
deliberate resistance by peasants. In 1960, Edgar Snow, visiting a

rural clinic in Sichuan, heard that the number of requests for information was 'light'.[15]

Jan Myrdal provides us with an interesting first-hand account from a village in Shaanxi in 1962. His interviewee, a thirty-two-year-old mother of three and head of a women's organisation, explained the difficulties encountered in the campaign:

Birth control is primarily a matter of propaganda. Firstly, many say: 'We want to have more children'; secondly, after all birth control is voluntary. We have discussed which contraceptives are best. Personally, I find the condom to be the most reliable. They are rather inexpensive too: thirty-three for one yuan. But there are other methods, too, and certain of the families don't use any contraceptives at all but only simple techniques. A lot of women still believe that they can't become with child as long as they are suckling. And each time, they are as surprised as ever, when they find they are pregnant again. But we are working to enlighten them.

In certain families with lots of children, the women would like birth control, but their husbands won't. In those families the husbands say: 'There's not going to be any family planning here!' Then we women go to them and try to talk sense to them. We say: 'Look how many children you have. Your wife looks after the household and sees to all the children and she makes shoes and clothes for both you and the children, but you don't think of all she has to do or of her health, but just make her with child again and again. Wait now for three or four years. Then you can have more if you want.' Usually, they will eventually say: 'If it isn't going to go on all one's life, then all right. But if she's going to go on with birth control for ever, then I'm not having any.' In those cases, all goes well and usually they do not decide to have any more afterwards. But in other cases, the husband just says: 'No.' Then we women speak to him about it every day, till he agrees to birth control. No husband has yet managed to stand out for any length of time, when we are talking to him. Actually, of course, they know that we are right. They know, of course, that they are responsible. It's only their pride that stands in the way, and we have to tell them that such pride is false and not at all right. But there are, too, families, where both husband and wife are agreed that they want to have children all the time. We can't do anything there. The whole thing's voluntary. The chief thing is to have a healthy family, and that the mother feels all right.[16]

In addition to these reservations expressed by male peasants, there were not only the practical difficulties of implementing birth control over such a wide area but also, as Gilbert Etienne emphasises, the interruptions to the campaign itself resulting from changes in domestic policy.[17] In any event, Edgar Snow, noting the progress made in China, remarked to Mao Zedong in a 1970 interview that it seemed no-one was objecting any more to birth control. Snow said:

> According to Mao I had been taken in. He said that in the countryside if a woman's first child is a girl she wants to have a boy. If the second is a girl, again she wants to have a boy. The third one comes, a girl again, and she still tries for a boy. Soon there are nine of them, all are girls, by then she is already forty-five, so she can only leave it at that![18]

The celebrated 'barefoot doctors', who appeared in 1966, played an important role in the promotion of family planning in the countryside. One of them, a young woman of nineteen, informed Maria-Antonietta Macciocchi in 1970 that

> our centre has thirty-six barefoot doctors, two for each brigade, and we are split into two teams of eighteen. The first team is only women, aged nineteen to thirty, who also act as midwives and distribute contraceptive information. Women are more listened-to than men on the birth control question.

This propaganda, she added, 'is closely tied to ideology'.[19] Dr Pierre Rentchnick observed on his return to China in 1973 that 'a real climate of social and political persuasion had been created . . . aimed at achieving a more or less voluntary chastity among the people'.[20] In his book *La Vie Sexuelle en Chine Communiste* (*Sexual Life in Communist China*), Dr Georges Valensin made a similar observation: 'Whether liked or not, contraception, although not legally obligatory, had been imposed on people after the second child through persistent persuasion and advice; if contraception fails and a third pregnancy occurs, the couple are obliged to provide an explanation'.[21]

Edgar Snow remarked in 1970 that 'in China today all methods of birth control are being carried out on a large scale'. Other observers like Dr Pierre Rentchnick agreed. On the question of abortion, Rentchnick, citing a Japanese report, recalled in his book *Esculape dans la Chine de Mao* (*Medicine in Mao's China*) that it had been practised since 1957 in China, 'pioneer of the suction method'. He added that 'one could see the equipment for this type of operation in virtually all of the 70,000 commune hospitals'.[22] In answer to the question of whether China encouraged abortion as a contraceptive method at the beginning of the 1970s, Edgar Snow replied in the negative: 'It is usually a last resort for mothers of one or more children who have not received or succeeded with contraceptive devices'.[23]

Currently, the emphasis is on the 'one-child family'. An article published in a Hong Kong journal in 1985 takes issue with this policy, disagreeing with those 'who assume that a strict control of demographic growth in China is necessary for economic progress' and underlining the harmful psychological and moral effects of such a policy, one of which is female infanticide (supposedly prohibited by the Marriage Reform Law of 30 April 1950).[24]

Public Health

Calling on Communist Party members to be 'promoters of revolution', Mao Zedong during the course of a speech on 9 October 1957 broached the problem of hygiene:

> Then there is the question of eliminating the four pests and paying attention to hygiene. I'm very keen on wiping out the four pests – rats, sparrows, flies and mosquitos. As there are only ten years left, can't we make some preparations and carry out propaganda this year and set about the work next spring? Because that is just the time when flies emerge. I still think that we should wipe out these pests and that the whole nation should pay particular attention to hygiene. This is a question of civilization, the level of which should be significantly raised. There should be an emulation drive; every possible effort must be made to wipe out these pests and everyone should pay attention to hygiene.[25]

Given the appalling hygienic conditions under which most Chinese lived, Mao's sense of urgency was understandable. Strict preventive measures were imposed with the aim of eradicating infectious and parasitic diseases. During the 1950s, plague, cholera, smallpox and blackwater fever were gradually eliminated. Measures to combat malaria took a little longer to succeed, but in 1983 there were no more than 1,360,000 people affected by this disease,[26] a considerable improvement when one considers that more than 30,000,000 had been affected with it thirty years earlier. With regard to bilharzia, a parasitic disease widespread in China, the Minister of Public Health, Cui Yueli, announced in 1986 that it had completely disappeared in 56 of the 348 districts and towns where the disease had raged in 1950.[27] Dr Pierre Rentchnick observed with some validity that in the campaign against bilharzia 'the most important aspect was the education of the public, which for the most part wholeheartedly participated in the effort to eradicate from certain regions the snails at the origin of the disease'.[28] Edgar Snow also cites a 1957 report by a British academic, Brian Maegraith, who emphasised 'the degree of general cooperation obtained from the people'.[29] On 1 July 1958, Mao Zedong, delighted by the news that a district in the south had succeeded in eradicating bilharzia, composed a poem entitled 'Farewell to the God of Plagues':

> The waters and hills displayed their green in vain
> When the ablest physicians were baffled by these pests.
> A thousand villages were overrun by brambles and men
>   were feeble;
> Ghosts sang their ballads in a myriad desolate houses.
> Now, in a day, we have leapt around the earth
> And inspected a thousand Milky Ways.
> If the Cowherd asks about the god of plagues,
> Tell him that with joy and sorrow he has been washed
>   away by the tide.[30]

The journal *China Reconstructs* reported in 1985 that in Dali (Yunnan province) 'thirty-two years of effort had resulted in halting the progress of bilharzia and saving 235,000 victims'. The report continued that 'as a consequence, out of eleven districts hit by bilharzia, six had virtually been cleared . . . the tragic scenes of rotting corpses in the household and the living pitifully grieving, houses in a state of collapse and fields being swallowed up by weeds . . . have ended'. In this area, the 'God of Plagues' had been expelled, but only after the most persistent effort: 'Since the end of the 1950s, the inhabitants of Dali, emulating other affected regions, have mobilized their resources in the destruction of the snails'.[31]

In 1986, after thirty-five years of effort to prevent and control leprosy, the number of lepers in China was estimated at 100,000. Thus in the province of Shandong the rate of leprosy fell from 5.07 per 100,000 inhabitants in the years 1955–9 to 0.14 from 1980–4. Throughout the country, more than 10,000 specialists in the disease were trained and over 1,100 leper clinics were opened. A research centre for the control of leprosy was created, while the Chinese Association for the Prevention and Treatment of Leprosy was founded under the direction of Dr Ma Haide. In 1985, an international symposium on leprosy was held in Guangzhou. Finally, research was especially carried out on a plant of the celastraceae family, *Tripterygium wilfordii*, considered 'effective in halting the onset of leprosy'.[32]

During the 1950s, tuberculosis was still a principal cause of death. Anti-TB vaccinations were introduced, and by 1958

17,000,000 had been vaccinated. The mortality rate due to tuberculosis fell from 230 per 100,000 in 1949 to 46 per 100,000 in 1958. Several vaccination campaigns against poliomyelitis were also carried out, and in 1973 Dr Pierre Rentchnick could affirm that 'the People's Republic has equalled the West in the control of poliomyelitis'.[33] Another victory for Chinese medicine was the eradication of venereal disease. One person in particular who played a key role in this campaign was Dr Ma Haide, who directed the Central Institute for Research into Skin and Venereal Diseases. The task was not easy. In 1972, Ma Haide confided to his Swiss colleague, Pierre Rentchnick, that 'as it was not possible to carry out blood tests on the entire population, a way had to be found to track down those carrying the disease, perhaps one out of 100 or 1,000 people'. A questionnaire to reveal hidden cases was tried out first in Hubei, and then in Jiangxi from 1958. The population was mobilised: '3,000 volunteers learned how to carry out blood tests and to vaccinate positive cases with penicillin injections; in two months they tracked down 49,000 suspected cases'.[34]

The Minister of Public Health, Cui Yueli, was pleased to note in 1986 that 'the major cause of death was no longer due to infectious and parasitic diseases but rather to brain haemorrhages, heart problems and malignant tumors'.[35] Although the battle against cancer remains the top priority towards the end of the twentieth century, doctors in the People's Republic have been preoccupied with the problem for some time. One of the most significant figures in Chinese cancer research has been Professor Wu Huanxing. A former student of Shanghai's Aurore University, Wu became head of the Shanghai Sino-Belgian Institute of Radiotherapy in 1946 after visiting London and Brussels. In 1958, he was appointed director of a newly-opened hospital in Beijing that specialised in the treatment of cancerous tumours; in 1963 he became head of the Institute of Cancer Research. Wu is the author of numerous works, and he enjoys an international reputation.

The Institute for Cancer Research has carried out extensive work on cancer of both the oesophagus and liver; in addition to its research and investigative work, the Institute has played an important role since its foundation in the training of specialists, doctors and hospital workers. Moreover, the battle against cancer has been specifically mentioned in the sixth Five-Year Plan (1981–5) as one of the key objectives of public health. In 1984, Wu Huanxing remarked to a Chinese journalist that

> since Liberation China has made rapid progress . . . over twenty specialized hospitals have been established in different regions.

With regard to pharmacological research into cancer, a high level has been attained. Various clinical experiments prove that fifty-six varieties of medicine tried out by Chinese specialists have a certain efficacy in combating malignant tumors.[36]

An example of the progress made is provided by the research of Zeng Yi, whose method of 'immuno-adsorption of linked enzymes' facilitates the early diagnosis of nose and throat cancer.[37]

This brief overview does not do justice to all the achievements in the medical field since 1949, but some others should be mentioned, such as the first reattachment of a severed hand in 1963 by the pioneer of Chinese microsurgery, Chen Zhongwei. Psychiatry also deserves mention. It has been noted that 'in 1950 the number of beds available in psychiatric wards represented 1.1 per cent of the total number of hospital beds; by 1957 the figure was 3.6 per cent. In 1958 the number of doctors in psychiatric hospitals was sixteen times more than in 1949, while the number of nurses was twenty times more numerous.'[38] Psychiatric facilities expanded considerably from the late 1950s on, and in 1982 a city such as Shanghai had 5,300 beds in various psychiatric establishments compared to 400 before 1949.[39]

Special measures were also taken to ensure the health of elderly people. Geriatric services were provided in all hospitals, while in 1964 the first National Conference on Geriatrics took place in Beijing.

The gradual improvement of health conditions in China after 1949 was accompanied by the creation of an infrastructure of health protection. Priority has been given since 1949 to preventive medicine, one of the three objectives adopted by the first National Conference on Public Health held in Beijing on 7 August 1950: all 'health work' (*weisheng gongzuo*) had to be 'aimed at workers, peasants and soldiers' (*mianxiang gong, nong, bing*), prevention was to be considered 'essential' (*yufang wei zhu*), and 'Chinese and western medicine were to be combined' (*tuanjie zhongxiyi*). The most urgent task was to create an appropriate hospital network. In 1952, there were 139,000 beds in public hospitals, an increase of 135 per cent compared to 1951 and 217 per cent compared to 1950. The number of beds exceeded 154,000 in 1953.[40] An indication of the progress made is shown by the fact that in 1981 the country possessed 951,510 hospital beds, that is to say fifteen times more than in 1949 (when the number was 63,767).[41]

These figures concern the important urban centres, but from 1965 the Ministry of Public Health concentrated its efforts on the countryside in line with Mao Zedong's call to 'put the emphasis on health and medical work in the rural areas.' The following personal testimony of a production brigade doctor, as reported by Jan Myrdal in his study of a Chinese village in 1969, suggests that such an emphasis had previously been lacking: 'We understood Chairman Mao's call to take power in the domains of medicine and health . . . It was not convenient to see a doctor in town. People had to queue and even then they were not well cared for.' Citing the case of one of his patients, the doctor added that 'he spent thirty entire working days waiting to see a doctor . . . if he needs to be treated again he can now come here'.[42]

This testimony illustrated the need to establish permanent health care in the countryside. The most innovative measure taken was to train a corps of peasant-physicians capable of treating everyday illnesses. A Chinese doctor explained to Maria-Antonietta Macciocchi in 1970 that 'they do not stop working in the commune, they simply divide their time between medicine and the soil. They are also the living proof that a doctor's work is not totally apart from other people's.'[43] These peasant-physicians were to be known as 'barefoot doctors' and by 1984 totalled 1,280,000 in number.[44] At the same time, an infrastructure of health care was either expanded or created. By the early 1980s, there were 2,829 district hospitals (326,000 beds), 55,000 township hospitals (763,114 beds) and 610,000 dispensaries, in addition to a variety of specialised establishments (to combat epidemics, for example),[45] among which particular mention must be made of health schools because of their role in the training, or perfecting the skills, of barefoot doctors.

University-level medical instruction was adversely affected by the Cultural Revolution, and in 1970 the period of study was reduced from six to three years. Lin Biao and the Gang of Four were later to be accused of destroying medical education (principally with regard to shortening the period of study), 'bringing untold harm to the younger generation'.[46]

The Same Struggle to Combine Chinese and Western Medicine

The blending of Chinese and western medicine was one of the aims laid down by the 1950 National Conference on Health in Beijing. For this to be achieved, traditional Chinese medicine had to attain a level of development that would render it credible. Edgar Snow, for example, remarked that he 'considered empirical Chinese medicine genuine quackery, as did most foreigners'.[47] A new confidence needed also to be given to practitioners of Chinese medicine by associating them with the collective effort to improve health. In this way, they were bestowed a 'legal' status. Training courses were organised to acquaint them with both modern methods and a scientific approach towards traditional Chinese medicine. The opening of traditional hospitals was encouraged; according to figures provided in 1986 by Cui Yueli, the Minister of Public Health, such hospitals totalled only 171 in 1976, but by 1983 exceeded 1,200.[48] Measures were also taken to encourage the teaching of traditional medicine, which formed an integral component of the medical curriculum. Special effort was made to improve the quality of plant-based medicines, the industrial production of which was gradually modernised. In a document published in 1983 by the World Health Organisation, Wang Pei, director of the Central Laboratory of the Academy of Traditional Chinese Medicine, emphasised that research activity had led to some 'encouraging' results. These concerned not only the fields of acupuncture and its use as an analgesic, back and joint injuries and cardiovascular illness, but also 'the hypotheses on which traditional medicine is based'.[49]

Analgesia by acupuncture was without doubt one of the most spectacular results of the policy to combine Chinese and western medicine. At the beginning of the 1970s, such a practice was referred to as a 'victory for Mao Zedong thought',[50] although Edgar Snow observed cautiously that 'enthusiasm for the therapeutic benefits of . . . acupuncture should be kept within bounds'.[51] Moreover, Pierre Rentchnick, replying to those who were incorrectly using the word 'anaesthesia', noted that 'acupuncture has never been used to induce a general or local anaesthesia'.[52] In any event, it was calculated that at the beginning of the 1980s 'fifteen to twenty per cent of all surgical operations (in the People's Republic) were carried out under analgesia induced by acupuncture'.[53] Research was also undertaken to find out more about the analgesic effects of acupuncture.

'The same struggle goes on to combine Chinese and western medicine.' Although such a slogan never appeared in Beijing, Shanghai or Guangzhou, it perfectly illustrated the spirit behind the health policy carried out in the People's Republic from its inception in 1949. Maria-Antonietta Macciocchi heard it said in 1970 that 'the fusion of western and Chinese medicine is a shining idea of Mao's'.[54] Alain Peyrefitte, for his part, observed in 1973 that western medicine had been incorporated into Chinese medicine 'without dominating or replacing it'.[55] It was within this context, for example, that a method was perfected for treating fractures and eliminating for the most part subsequent complications (e.g. ankylosis and

muscular atrophy). Such a treatment, explained an orthopaedist
and traumatologist,

> allows for both movement and securing the fracture against
> motion, involving the use of small wooden splints attached to
> the outside of the body, the setting of the fracture by the
> surgeon, and the active participation of the patient, who is
> encouraged to perform functional exercises. The clinical
> recovery period is reduced by one-third, while the total period
> of treatment is reduced by one-half.[56]

The combination of the two medical traditions was put into
practice in other areas, notably in those of preventive medicine and
hygiene. Thus in 1974 a prophylactic exercise, relying on the
massage of acupuncture points, was tried out to ward off colds.[57] A
similar method was even devised to treat Ménière's syndrome
(disease of the membranous labyrinth of the ear).[58] Traditional
practices, moreover, were given new credence. One such practice
was that of *huanghai*, which consisted of being in a seated position
with hands on knees and the head and back erect, then moving the
trunk in a circular fashion from right to left. The exercise, which is
especially recommended for insomnia,[59] requires the person to do
this thirty-six times and then to repeat the action thirty-six times
from left to right. The benefits of traditional gymnastic exercises,
such as *taijiquan*, were once again recognised, not only in
strengthening the body but also to prevent and even cure various
chronic illnesses.

Referring to China's medical and pharmacological legacy, Mao
Zedong declared that 'we must strive to explore it fully and raise it
to a higher level'. Encouraged by this exhortation, Chinese
researchers (one of whose most notable successes was to produce
synthetic insulin in 1965) did not hesitate to follow in the footsteps
of their illustrious predecessors, Li Shizhen (sixteenth century) and
Zhao Xuemin (eighteenth century), and make use of the 4,000–
5,000 medicinal plants growing in China, 1,000 of which are
commonly used in traditional medicine. Chemical, pharmacological
and clinical research carried out since 1949 has led to the discovery
of many new substances whose beneficial physiological effects
have been demonstrated. The tranquillising, sedative, analgesic
and even anaesthetic properties of certain Chinese drugs have
been known for a long time, but Hua Tuo, for example, in the
second century, was unaware that the analgesic he used owed its
efficacy to the action of scopolamine. Significantly, popular tradition
in Tibet and Qinghai has preserved the use of a solanaceous plant,

Scopolia tangutica (*Anisodus tanguticus*), as an analgesic.[60]

The struggle against parasitic diseases has benefited from important discoveries. Artemisinin, the extract from the artemisia (*qinghaosu* in Chinese), for example, has been shown to be effective against malaria. The cardiovascular system has also attracted the attention of Chinese researchers, who have taken an interest in the use of sage (*Salvia miltiorrhiza*), referred to as 'red root' (*danshen*) in traditional materia medica. It has been used as a tonic since the appearance of the *Shen'nong Bencaojing*, and one of its active elements (tanshinone) is used to treat angina and coronary thrombosis. In treating cancer, the simultaneous use of chemotherapy and phytotherapy (to enhance the body's immunity) has led to a study of the active elements of traditional drugs, for example the fruit of a tree belonging to the family of Nyssaceae, *Camptotheca acuminata*, the alkaloid extract of which has therapeutic benefits for certain cancers (particularly cancer of the liver).

With a population exceeding one billion, the People's Republic, as was noted earlier, has been compelled to adopt draconian birth-control measures for a society that has traditionally set great store by large families. Traditional materia medica refer to the abortive and emmenagogic properties of numerous drugs (Li Shizhen, in his *Bencao Gangmu*, described twenty-seven drugs as abortive and ninety-seven as emmenagogues). Research focused particularly on the drugs mentioned by Li Shizhen, and the results were encouraging. For example, Li Shizhen had noted the abortive properties of *Daphne genkwa*. It has been proved that the root extract of this plant (*yuanhua* in Chinese) increases the number of uterine contractions. Chinese researchers have also extracted a polypeptide (trichosanthin) from the tuberous root of a cucurbitaceous plant (*Trichosanthes kirilowii*) which was used in conjunction with six other traditional plants to induce abortion. The abortive properties of this polypeptide (whose composition has been analysed by X-ray) have been demonstrated. Furthermore, it was brought to light in the 1960s that male sterility caused by cottonseed oil was due to the action of gossypol, a toxic phenolic crystalline compound. This discovery gave a new impetus to research on male contraceptives.

'Much work remains to be done', modestly concluded three researchers from the Shanghai Institute of Materia Medica in a 1985 report on recent research into Chinese medicinal plants. They added: 'There are now numerous scientists and institutions engaged in such research, and the technical facilities are constantly being improved. It is therefore certain that a great deal of useful information will become available in the very near future.'[61]

Notes

1. Jacques Guillermaz, *The Chinese Communist Party in Power 1949–1976* (Boulder: Westview Press, 1976), p 3.
2. Mao Zedong, 'Fight for a Fundamental Turn for the Better in the Nation's Financial and Economic Situation' (6 June 1950), *Selected Works of Mao Tsetung*, vol. 5 (Peking: Foreign Language Press, 1977), pp 26–32.
3. Gilbert Etienne, *La Voie Chinoise* (Paris: PUF, 1974), p 57.
4. Mao Zedong, 'On the Co-operative Transformation of Agriculture' (31 July 1955), *Selected Works of Mao Tsetung*, vol. 5, p 184.
5. Edgar Snow, *The Long Revolution* (London: Hutchinson, 1973), p 68.
6. K. S. Karol, *La Deuxième Revolution Chinoise* (Paris: Robert Laffont, 1973).
7. Maria-Antonettia Macciocchi, *Daily Life in Revolutionary China* (New York: Monthly Review Press, 1972).
8. Simon Leys, *Les Habits Neufs du Président Mao* (Paris: Editions Champ Libre, 1971), p 23.
9. Han Suyin, *Wind in the Tower* (London: Jonathan Cape, 1976), p 390.
10. Jacques Guillermaz, *The Chinese Communist Party in Power 1949–1976*, p 158.
11. Mao Zedong, 'Be Activists in Promoting the Revolution' (9 October 1957), *Selected Works of Mao Tsetung*, vol. 5, p 488.
12. Mao Zedong, 'Have Firm Faith in the Majority of the People' (13 October 1957), *Selected Works of Mao Tsetung*, vol. 5, p 512.
13. Edgar Snow, *The Other Side of the River* (London: Victor Gollancz, 1963), p 413.
14. Alain Peyrefitte, *Quand la Chine s'éveillera* (Paris: Fayard, 1973), p 282.
15. Edgar Snow, *The Other Side of the River*, p 414.
16. Jan Myrdal, *Report from a Chinese Village*, pp 226–7.
17. Gilbert Etienne, *La Voie Chinoise*, op. cit., p 76.
18. Edgar Snow, *The Long Revolution*, p 44.
19. Maria-Antonietta Macciocchi, *Daily Life in Revolutionary China*, p 290.
20. Pierre Rentchnick, *Esculape dans la Chine de Mao* (Geneva: Editions Médecine et Hygiène, 1973), p 128.
21. Georges Valensin, *La Vie Sexuelle en Chine Communiste* (Paris: Edition J. C. Lattès, 1977), p 83.
22. Pierre Rentchnick, op. cit., p 132.
23. Edgar Snow, *The Long Revolution*, p 33.
24. *Jiushiniandai*, no 189, cited in *Bulletin de Sinologie* (Hong Kong: French Cultural Service), no 10, pp 7–8.
25. Mao Zedong, 'Be Activists in Promoting the Revolution' (9 October 1957), *Selected Works of Mao Tsetung*, vol. 5, p 488.
26. Ding Youhe and Luo Yiqin, 'Public health", *China Reconstructs*, no 7 (1984), p 6.
27. Cui Yueli, 'Developing medical and health services', *China Reconstructs*, no 2 (1986), p 25.
28. Pierre Rentchnick, op. cit., p 103.
29. Edgar Snow, *The Other Side of the River*, p. 305.

30. Translated in J. Ch'en, *Mao and the Chinese Revolution* (Oxford: Oxford University Press, 1965), p 349.
31. Deng Shulin, *China Reconstructs*, no 12 (1985), pp 43–5.
32. Deng Shulin, *China Reconstructs*, no 6 (1986), pp 20–3. The active elements of *Tripterygium wilfordii* have been isolated. Two triterpene triepoxides, tripdiolide and triptolide, have been shown to have anti-leukaemia properties. These derivatives are currently produced through tissue culture. See Misawa, Hayashi and Takayama, *Planta medica*, 49:2 (1983), pp 115–19.
33. Pierre Rentchnick, op. cit., p 102.
34. Pierre Rentchnick, op. cit., pp 92–100.
35. *China Reconstructs*, no 2 (1986), p 25.
36. *China Reconstructs*, no 4 (1984), p 45.
37. Ma Xiaoquan, 'A Specialist in Nose and Throat Cancer', *China Reconstructs*, no 7 (1986), p 39.
38. Gregorio Bermann, *La Santé Mentale en Chine* (Paris: Editions François Maspero, 1973), p 84.
39. 'Treatment of Mental Illness in Shanghai', *China Reconstructs*, no 2 (1982), p 40.
40. Yu Shenchu, *Zhongguo Yixue Jianshi*, op. cit., p 440.
41. *China Reconstructs*, no 10 (1982), p 10. Edgar Snow, *The Other Side of the River*, p 304, notes that in 1960 there were '1,200 hospitals with 467,000 beds, as distinct from about 200,000 clinics and health stations in the rural communes'. Gregorio Bermann gives the same figures in *La Santé Mentale en Chine*, op. cit., p 17, while adding: 'Gradually the country approached the necessary minimum number of hospitals'.
42. Jan Myrdal, *Un Village de la Chine Populaire* (Paris: Gallimard, 1972), p 443.
43. Maria-Antonietta Macciocchi, *Daily Life in Revolutionary China*, pp 282–3.
44. *China Reconstructs*, no 7 (1984), p 8.
45. *China Reconstructs*, no 10 (1982), pp 10, 11.
46. Huang Jiasi, 'Development of Surgery in China in the Last Fifteen Years', *Chinese Medical Journal*, no 1 (1979) p 6.
47. Edgar Snow, *The Long Revolution*, p 35.
48. *China Reconstructs*, no 2 (1986), p 26.
49. Wang Pei, *Médecine Chinoise Traditionnelle*, op. cit., p 73.
50. Alain Peyrefitte, op. cit., pp 78–82.
51. Edgar Snow, *The Long Revolution*, p 40.
52. Pierre Rentchnick, op. cit., p 90.
53. 'Acupuncture and Moxibustion', *Médecine Traditionnelle et Couverture des Soins de Santé*, op. cit., pp 79, 80.
54. Maria-Antonietta Macciocchi, *Daily Life in Revolutionary China*, p 278.
55. Alain Peyrefitte, op. cit., p 82.
56. Shang Tianyu, 'Traitement des fractures et des lésions des tissus mous par des méthodes combinant la médecine chinoise traditionnelle et la médecine occidentale' (Treatment of fractures and lesions of soft tissue by methods combining traditional Chinese medicine with western medicine), *Médecine Traditionnelle et Couverture des Soins de Santé*, op. cit., p 86.
57. 'The Gymnastic Exercise to Prevent Cold', *China Reconstructs*, no 3 (1982), pp 10–12.

58. 'Treatment of Ménière's Syndrome', *China Reconstructs*, no 4 (1984), p 23.
59. 'The *huanghai*', *China Reconstructs*, no 6 (1984), p 60. 'Throughout the exercise the person must try to think of the sky or the sea, imagining that he or she is in the middle of a vast open space.'
60. Pharmacological study of two alkaloids containing tropane extracted from the *Scopolia tangutica*, anisodamine and anisodine, has revealed they have an antispasmodic effect similar to that of atropine. See Xiao Peigen and He Liyi, 'Ethnopharmacologic Investigation on Tropane-containing Drugs in Chinese Solanaceous Plants', *Journal of Ethnopharmacology*, no 8 (1983), pp 1–18.
61. Xu Renshang, Zhu Qiaozhen and Xie Yuyuan, 'Recent Advances in Studies on Chinese Medicinal Herbs with Physiological Activity', *Journal of Ethnopharmacology*, no 14 (1985), pp 222–53. On gossypol, see Yun Cheung Kong, Jingxi Xie and Paul Pui-Hay But, 'Fertility-regulating Agents from Traditional Chinese Medicines', *Journal of Ethnopharmacology*, no 15 (1986), pp 1–44.

Appendices

Chronology of Chinese Medicine

Seventeenth to eleventh centuries BC Oracle-bone inscriptions (e.g. 'Is the king going to suffer from a toothache?'). Discovery at Taixi in 1973 of fruit-stones of the *Prunus persica* and *Prunus japonica*, and of a medical instrument known as *bian*.

Eleventh to eighth centuries BC The *Shijing* (*Book of Odes*) and *Shanhaijing* (*Classic of Mountains and Seas*) list numerous drugs of plant, mineral and animal origin used at the time. According to the *Zhouli* (*Rites of Zhou*), internal medicine was already being distinguished from external medicine.

Eighth to third centuries BC Development of the theory of meridians (channels), of which the earliest mention is to be found in the *Zhubi Shiyi Mai Jiujing* and the *Yinyang Shiyi Mai Jiujing* discovered at Mawangdui. Compilation of the *Huangdi Neijing* (*Yellow Emperor's Classic of Internal Medicine*).

Fourth century BC Qin Yueren (Bian Que) establishes the diagnostic procedures of Chinese medicine.

Second century BC Chunyu Yi records his clinical observations.

First century BC Compilation of *Shen'nong Bencaojing* (*Shen'nong's Classic of Herbal Medicine*).

Second century AD Zhang Zhongjing compiles the *Shanghanlun*. Hua Tuo pioneers the use of an anaesthetic drug and devises a gymnastic exercise known as 'the five animals'.

Third century AD Wang Shuhe promotes the technique of pulsing. Huangfu Mi brings together all previous knowledge in the domain of acupuncture and compiles the *Zhenjiu Jiayijing* (*ABC of Acupuncture and Moxibustion*).

Fourth century AD Ge Hong, alchemist and physician, compiles the *Zhouhou Beijifang* (*Emergency Prescriptions*).,

Fifth century AD Compilation of the *Lei Gong Baozhilun* (*Treatise on the Preparation of Lei Gong's Remedies*). Gong Qingxuan compiles the *Liu Juanzi Guiyifang*, the earliest treatise on surgery in China.

c. 500 AD Tao Hongjing revises and annotates the *Shen'nong Bencaojing*.

Sixth century AD A hundred prescriptions are engraved in a cave at Longmen, near Luoyang.

Seventh century AD Chao Yuanfang writes the *Zhubing Yuanhoulun* (*Treatise on the Causes and Symptoms of Illnesses*).

641 Through marriage, the Chinese princess Wencheng contributes to the diffusion of Chinese medical works in Tibet.

659 Su Jing completes the *Xinxiu Bencao* (*Newly-revised Materia Medica*).

581–682 Sun Simiao, author of the *Qianjin Yaofang* (*Prescriptions of the Thousand Ounces of Gold*), defines the ideal physician, establishes himself as a phytotherapist, focuses on deficiency-related illnesses, and champions the health of mother and child.

713–41 Chen Cangqi completes previous materia medica with his *Bencao Shiyi*.

752 Wang Tao completes his summary on medicine, the *Waitai Miyao*, and advocates protection for the pregnant woman.

753–63 The Buddhist monk Jianzhen takes to Japan his medical and pharmaceutical knowledge.

852–6 Zan Yin completes the *Chanbao* (*Treasure of Childbirth*), the first Chinese work on gynaecology and obstetrics.

Eighth and ninth centuries Alchemy reaches the Arab world.

974 Compilation of the *Kaibao Chongding Bencao* (*Revised Materia Medica of the Kaibao Era*).

982–92 Wang Huaiyin oversees the compilation of medical prescriptions collectively known as the *Taiping Shenghuifang*.

1026 Wang Weiyi writes the *Tongren Shuxue Zhenjiu Tujing* (*Illustrated Manual of the Bronze Man Showing Acupuncture and Moxibustion Points*).

1061 Compilation of the *Jiayou Buzhou Shen'nong Bencaojing* (*Complete and Annotated Classic of Herbal Medicine of the Jiayou Era*). Su Song compiles the *Tujing Bencao* (*Illustrated Materia Medica*).

1075 Compilation of the *Su Shen Liangfang* (*Efficacious Prescriptions of Su and Shen*).

1082 Tang Shenwei writes his *Zhenglei Bencao* (*Classified Materia Medica*).

1086 Han Zhihe writes *Shanghan Weizhi* (*Hidden Meanings of Shanghan Illnesses*).

1093 Dong Ji discusses smallpox among children in *Xiao'er Banzhen Beiji Fanglun*.

1098 The obstetrician Yang Zijian describes for the first time the 'version' method in his *Shichanlun*.

1100 Pang Anshi compiles the *Shanghan Zongbinglun* (*General Treatise on Shanghan Illnesses*).

1102–6 Yang Jie publishes in the *Cunzhentu* anatomical drawings based on dissections carried out on executed prisoners.

1107 Chen Shiwen compiles the *Hejijufang* (*Prescriptions from the Pharmacy of Harmonious Assistance*). Zhu Gong completes the *Nanyang Huorenshu*.

1111–17 Compilation of the *Shengji Zonglu* (*General Catalogue of Divine Assistance*).

1116 Kou Zongshi publishes the *Bencao Yanyi* (*Development of Herbal Medicine*).

1119 Yan Xiaozhang records Qian Yi's experiences in paediatrics in the

Xiao'er Yaozheng Zhijue (*The Appropriate Way of Recognising and Treating Infant Maladies*).

1132 Xu Shuwei publishes the *Puji Benshifang* (*Effective Prescriptions for the Relief of All*). Liu Fang publishes a summary of infant illnesses, the *Youyou Xinshu* (*New Book on Children*).

1144 Cheng Wuji produces an annotated version of the *Shanghanlun* (*Zhujie Shanghanlun*).

1156 Publication of the *Xiao'er Weisheng Zongwei Lunfang*.

1174 Chen Yan promulgates the theory of the 'three causes' in the *Sanyin Jiyi Bingzheng Fanglun*.

1182 Liu Wansu, founder of the Hejian School, outlines his pathogenic concepts in the *Suwen Xuanji Yuanbingshi*.

1184 Zhu Duanzhang publishes a treatise on obstetrics, *Weisheng Jiabao Chanke Beiyao*.

1186 Zhang Yuansu, master of the Yishui School, publishes his *Yixue Qiyuan* (*Explanation of Medicine*).

1189 Cui Jiayan publishes *Cuishi Maijue* (*Principles of the Pulse by Master Cui*). Zhang Gao writes the earliest text (still extant) on the history of Chinese medicine, the *Yishuo*.

1217–20 Zhang Congzheng writes the *Rumen Shiqin* and defends his theory of the 'six doors' and 'three methods'.

1220 Publication of Wang Zhizhong's summary of acupuncture and moxibustion, the *Zhenjiu Zishengjing*.

1226 Wenren Qinian writes a treatise on moxibustion, the *Beiji Jiufa*.

1236 Wang Haogu discusses the *yin* syndrome in *Yinzheng Lueli*.

1237 Chen Ziming writes the *Furen Daquan Liangfang*.

1241 Chen Wenzhong, author of the *Xiao'er Bingyuan Fanglun*, discusses smallpox among children in *Xiao'er Douzhen Fanglun*.

1247 Li Gao writes the *Neiwaishang Bianhuolun* (*Treatise on the Differentiation Between Endogenous and Exogenous Diseases*). Song Ci publishes a treatise on forensic medicine, the *Xiyuan Jilu*.

1249 Li Gao writes the *Piweilun* (*Treatise on the Spleen and Stomach*).

1253 Yan Yonghe compiles the *Jishengfang* (*Prescriptions to Save Life*).

1263 Chen Ziming publishes the *Waike Jingyao* (*Essentials of Surgery*).

1294 The paediatrician, Zeng Shirong, lists 230 remedies to treat infant illnesses in *Houyou Xinshu*.

1306 Wang Haogu publishes the *Tangye Bencao*.

1311 Dou Guifang publishes the *Zhenjiu Sishu* (*Four Books on Acupuncture and Moxibustion*).

1330 The Mongol, Hu Sihui, publishes the *Yinshan Zhengyao* (*Important Principles of Food and Drink*).

1335 Qi Dezhi suggests 145 remedies to treat skin disorders in the *Waike Jingyi* (*Essentials of External Medicine*).

1343 Wei Yilin compiles the *Shiyi Dexiaofang* (*Efficacious Remedies of the Physicians*) especially to deal with fractures and dislocations.

1347 Zhu Zhenheng discusses in the *Gezhi Yulun* the theory of 'minister-fire' and the weakening of *yin* energy.

1368 Wang Lu recommends in the *Yijing Suhuiji* to 'go against the tide of accepted opinion on the medical classics' in order to rediscover their original meaning, and suggests that *wenbing* ('febrile disease') should not be treated in the same way as *shanghan* ('cold-induced illness').

1371–1401 Lou Quanshan compiles the *Yixue Gangmu* (*Compendium of Medicine*).

1408 Completion of the *Yongle Dadian* (*Great Dictionary of the Yongle Reign*).

1518 The birth of Li Shizhen.

1529 Gao Wu publishes the *Zhenjiu Juying* (*The Best of Acupuncture and Moxibustion*). Xue Ji writes the *Neike Zhaiyao* (*Summary of Internal Medicine*), the *Zhengti Leiyao* (*A Repertory of Traumatology*) and the *Kouchi Leiyao* (*A Repertory of Stomatology*).

1531 Wang Ji condemns the abuse of surgical instruments in the *Waike Lili*.

1556 Xu Chunfu writes the *Gujin Yitong* (*Synthesis of Past and Present Medicine*).

1564 Li Shizhen composes the *Binhu Maixue* (*Binhu's Study of the Pulse*).

1572 Li Shizhen composes the *Qijing Bamai Kao* (*An Examination of the Eight Extra Meridians*).

1575 Li Jianzhai publishes the *Yixue Rumen* (*Rudiments of Medicine*).

1587 Gong Tingxian writes the *Wanbing Huichun*.

1592 Fang Youzhi publishes a commentary on the *Shanghanlun*.

1593 Death of Li Shizhen.

1596 Publication of the *Bencao Gangmu* (*Compendium of Materia Medica*).

1601 Yang Jizhou writes the *Zhenjiu Dacheng* (*The Great Success of Acupuncture and Moxibustion*).

1604 Gong Yunlin composes the *Xiao'er Tuina Mizhi* (*Hidden Significance of Infant Massage*).

1602–8 Wang Kentang compiles the *Zhengzhi Zhunsheng*.

1617 Chen Shigong describes cancer of the lip and the breast in the *Waike Zhengzong*.

1620 Wu Zhiwang writes the *Jiyin Gangmu* (*A Synopsis of Female Illnesses*).

1624 Zhang Jiebin 'classifies' the *Huangdi Neijing* (*Yellow Emperor's Classic of Internal Medicine*).

1632 Chen Sicheng recommends the use of arsenic and mercury to treat syphilitic ulcers in the *Meichuang Milu* (*Secret writings on Putrid Ulcers*).

1640 Zhang Jiebin (Jingyue) criticises the theories of Liu Wansu and Zhu Zhenheng in the *Jingyue Quanshu* (*The Complete Work of Zhang Jiebin*).

1642 Wu Youxing points out in his treatise *Wenyilun* (*On Pestilence*) the specific features of *wenyi* (pestilence) and outlines the theory of 'excessive, or evil, influences' – pathogenic agents responsible for the spread of pestilence. Li Zhongzi writes the *Neijing Zhiyao* (*What is Necessary to Know about the* Huangdi Neijing).

1644 Fu Renyu writes the *Shenshi Yaohan* (*Precious Letter on Vision*).

1665 Qi Kun publishes the *Waike Dacheng* (*Great Success of External Medicine*).

1669 Ke Qin records his thoughts on the *Shanghanlun* (*Shanghanlun Laisuji*).

1672 Zhang Zhicong edits and comments on the *Huangdi Neijing* (*Huangdi Neijing Suwen Lingshu Jizhu*).

1684 Publication of the *Nuke Jinglun* by Xiao Xun.

1687 Publication of the *Yiguan* by Zhao Xianke, and the *Zhengzhi Huibu* by Li Yongcui.

1694 Wang Ang compiles the *Bencao Beiyao* (*Emergency Materia Medica*).

1695 Xia Ding publishes the *Youke Tiejing* (*Iron Mirror of Paediatrics*).

1698–1741 The Jesuit missionary Parrenin attempts to introduce western anatomy into China, and corresponds with European scholars on Chinese medicine.

1703 (15 February) The Jesuit de Fontaney describes how the Kangxi emperor was cured of a 'third attack of fever' by taking quinquina.

1722 Dai Tianzhang publishes the *Guangwenyilun* (*Treatise on Pestilence*).

1726 (11 May) The Jesuit d'Entrecolles describes the 'Chinese method of obtaining the smallpox virus for children'.

1727 Yu Maokun publishes the *Douke Jinjing Fujijie*, in which he indicates that variolation was first practised in China around the years 1567–72.

1732 Cheng Guopeng publishes the *Yixue Xinwu* (*An Understanding of Medicine*).

1740 Wang Weide publishes the *Waike Zhengzhi Quanshengji*.

1742 Wu Qian publishes the *Yizong Jinjian* (*Golden Mirror of Medicine*).

1746 Ye Tianshi writes the *Wenrelun* (*On Febrile Illnesses*).

1750 Chen Xiazheng publishes his work on paediatrics, the *Youyou Jicheng*.

1751 Publication of the *Yibian* by He Mengyao.

1757 Publication of the *Bencao Congxin* by Wu Yiluo.

1759 Xu Dachun compiles the *Shanghanlun Leifang* (*Classified Remedies of the* Shanghanlun). Zhao Xuemin records the teachings of itinerant physicians in the *Chuanya*.

1765 Zhao Xuemin completes his *Bencao Gangmu Shiyi* (*Compendium of Materia Medica*).

1794 Yu Lin focuses on 'eruptive epidemic diseases' in his *Yizhen Yide*.

1798 Wu Tang discusses *wenbing* in the *Wenbing Tiaobian*.

1805 Gao Bingjun publishes the *Yangke Xindeji* (*Results of the Study of Skin Diseases*).

1808 Qian Changxiu publishes his book on traumatology, the *Shangke Buyao*.

1827 Publication of *Fu Qingzhu Nuke* (*Gynaecology of Fu Qingzhu*) by Fu Shan.

1830 Wang Qingren revives Chinese anatomy with the publication of *Yilin Gaicuo* (*Errors Corrected from the Forest of Physicians*).

1852 Wang Mengying writes about febrile illnesses in the *Wenre Jingwei*.

1853–4 The Taiping Kingdom of Heavenly Peace in Nanjing bans alcohol, tobacco and opium.

1863 Fei Boxiong warns against abusive use of drugs in the *Yichun Shengyi.*

1865 Publication of Chen Xiuyuan's *Yishu Shiliuzhong* (*Sixteen Volumes on Medicine*).

1882 Lei Feng compiles his treatise on seasonal illnesses, the *Shibinglun.*

1884 Tang Zonghai publishes a treatise on blood disorders, *Xuezhenglun.*

1892 Zhu Peiwen compares Chinese and western medicine in the *Huoyang Zangxiang Yuezuan.* Tang Zonghai founds the 'school of Sino-Western convergence and intercourse' and outlines its precepts in the *Zhongxi Huitong Yijing Jingyi.*

1912 Wang Daxie urges the abandonment of traditional Chinese medicine.

1909–24 In the *Yixue Zhongzhong Canxi Lu*, Zhang Xichun speaks up for Sino-Western medical interaction.

1929 The Guomindang government places restrictions on traditional Chinese medicine.

1935 Chen Cunren publishes the *Zhongguo Yaoxue Dacidian* (*Chinese Pharmaceutical Encyclopaedia*).

1938–9 The Canadian, Norman Bethune, becomes physician to the Eighth Route Army.

1947 Plague epidemic in north-east China.

1950 (7 August) First national conference on health recommends 'the combining of Chinese and western medicine'.

1957 (9 October) Mao Zedong declares: 'The complete realization of family planning will be out of the question without the weight of society as a whole behind it, that is, without general consent and joint effort'.

1965 Mao Zedong recommends that health and medical work should concentrate on the countryside. Insulin is synthetically produced.

1966 'Barefoot doctors' make an appearance in the countryside.

1981–5 The battle against cancer is mentioned in the sixth Five-Year Plan as one of the objectives of public health.

1986 Cui Yueli, Minister of Public Health, notes that 'the major cause of death was no longer due to infectious and parasitic diseases but rather to brain haemorrhages, heart problems and malignant tumors'.

Medical Journals Published in the
People's Republic of China

The 1987 catalogue of the China International Book Trading Corporation (Guoji Shudian) lists ninety-six titles, of which twenty-six concern traditional Chinese medicine. Many of these journals are published under the aegis of the Chinese Society of Medicine (*Zhonghua Yixuehui*), such as the *China Medical Review* (*Zhonghua Yixue Zazhi*), the *China Surgical Review* (*Zhonghua Waike Zazhi*), the *China Paediatrics Review* (*Zhonghua Erke Zazhi*) and the *China Otorhinolaryngology Review* (*Zhonghua Er-bi-yanhouke Zazhi*). Others are published by universities or research institutions, such as the *Beijing University Journal of Medical Science* (*Beijing Yike Daxue Xuebao*), the *Shandong University Journal of Medical Science* (*Shandong Yike Daxue Xuebao*), the *Xi'an University Journal of Medical Science* (*Xi'an Yike Daxue Xuebao*) and *Ophthalmological Research* (*Yanke Yanjiu*), published by the Henan Institute of Ophthalmological Research. Several associations have their own publications: the *Pharmacy Journal* (*Yaoxue Xuebao*) is produced by the Chinese Society of Pharmacy, while the *China Pharmacological Journal* (*Zhongguo Yaoli Xuebao*) is produced by the Chinese Society of Pharmacology. There also exists the *Medical Review of the People's Liberation Army* (*Jiefangjun Yixue Zazhi*).

Traditional Chinese medicine is served by reviews published by various institutions and societies, among which are the *Review of Chinese Medicine* (*Zhongyi Zazhi*), *Chinese Acupuncture and Moxibustion* (*Zhongguo Zhenjiu*), *China Journal of Medicine and Pharmacy* (*Zhongguo Yiyao Xuebao*), *Beijing Chinese Medicine* (*Beijing Zhongyi*) and the *Review of the Association of Chinese and Western Medicine* (*Zhongxiyi Jiehe Zazhi*).

All of these reviews are in Chinese. Some give an English summary of major articles, and most of them contain at least one summary in English. Finally, the *Chinese Medical Journal* is published entirely in English.

History of Chinese Medicine
in Comic Strip

Hua Tuo (141–208) is as much a historical as a legendary figure, and his popularity has made him a hero of the comic strips. The following extract from one such comic strip recounts an episode in his life that is recorded in the *Houhanshu* (*History of the Later Han*):

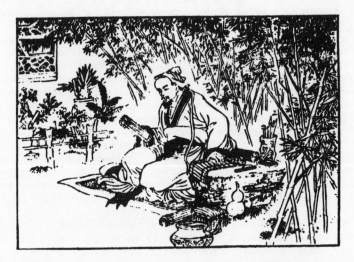

FIGURE A.1   Hua Tuo, the famous physician deeply loved by the people, lived during the Later Han dynasty and was a native of present-day Anhui province. Hua Tuo was thoroughly versed in medical theory, which he went to much trouble in studying in a conscientious and diligent way.

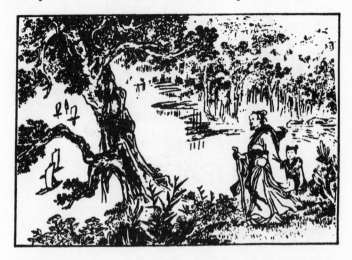

FIGURE A.2   In order to improve his medical knowledge, Hua Tuo
left his native village and travelled throughout the provinces of
Jiangsu and Shandong, all the while perfecting his knowledge and
practising medicine at the same time.

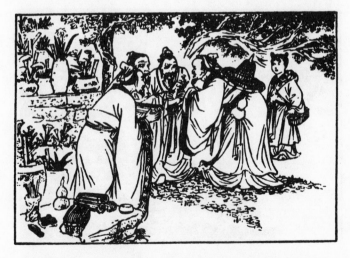

FIGURE A.3   At each place he stayed, Hua Tuo humbly sought
advice from local people and physicians. Thanks to his careful
questioning and his ability to summarise people's experiences,
Hua Tuo acquired a vast knowledge of popular medical practice.

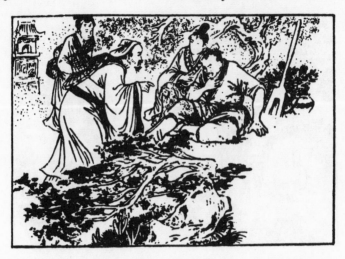

FIGURE A.4   Everywhere he went, Hua Tuo enthusiastically tended to the people's needs. One day he met an ailing man on the road. Hua Tuo approached him and asked what the trouble was. The man's throat was blocked, preventing him from swallowing and causing great pain.

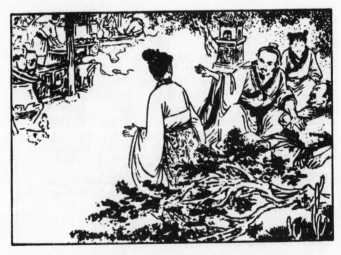

FIGURE A.5   After examining the man with great care, Hua Tuo concluded that a worm (helminth) was blocking the man's throat. He told him that all he needed to do was to buy some garlic from the store opposite, mix it with half a bowl of vinegar and drink it. He would then feel much better.

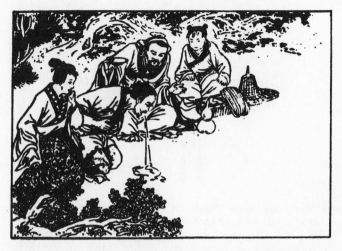

FIGURE A.6   After having drunk the garlic and vinegar, the man
vomited and expelled the worm. He then felt much better.

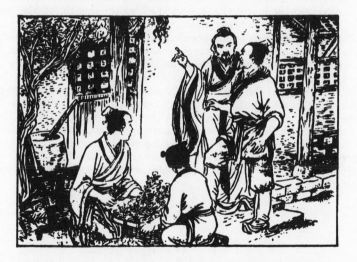

FIGURE A.7   As soon as he was cured, the man came to thank Hua
Tuo and discovered hanging on the wall of Hua Tuo's house more
than ten specimens of worm similar to the one he had vomited.
Hua Tuo, in fact, paid careful attention to parasitic diseases in his
research, and this is why his diagnosis and prescription were
correct.

From: *Hua Tuo* (Beijing: Renmin Meishu Chubanshu, 1979). Text
by Wang Zichun, drawings by Zhu Guangyu.

Medicine and Politics in the
People's Republic of China

One of Maria-Antonietta Macciocchi's interviewees in 1970, an elderly physician of seventy-three, expressed himself in these terms:

> All our research was aimed at making us physicians of renown in the great cities. Mao, on the contrary, teaches us that one must serve the poor peasants, the workers, and most of all those peasants who totally lack doctors. For years we did not follow Mao's line. Before the Cultural Revolution we were unaware of the weaknesses in our behaviour, even ethically. But in studying the thought of Mao we realized that we had been following a revisionist line.[1]

A dictionary of philosophy, published in Beijing in 1974, defined revisionism as 'a form of opportunism that waves the Marxist flag to oppose Marxism'.[2]

A comic strip designed to promote criticism of revisionism in the medical field, and published in 1976 shortly after the death of Mao Zedong and the fall of the 'Gang of Four', contrasts the attitudes of two physicians faced with a young peasant afflicted with chondrosarcoma (a kind of malignant tumour). The action takes place in the province of Yunnan. One of the physicians, Qian Bin, recommends amputating the arm: 'It's a malignant tumour, only an amputation can save his life'. The other, Jiang Hao, opposes this view and suggests carrying out an operation that would keep the arm intact. After a lengthy discussion, it is decided to perform the operation.

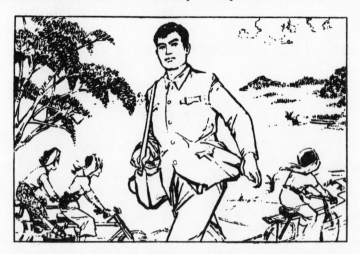

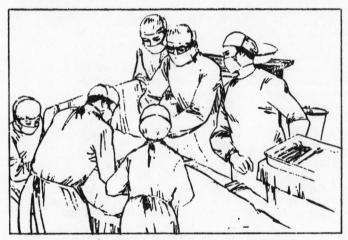

FIGURE A.8   From *Yiliao Duiyuan Zhi Ge* (*The Song of the Members of the Health Team*) (Shanghai: Shanghai Renmin Chubanshe, 1976).

Notes

1. Maria-Antonietta Macciocchi, *Daily Life in Revolutionary China*, p 271.
2. *Zhexue Mingci Jieshi* (Beijing: Renmin Chubanshe, 1974).

Index of Persons

Index of Plants